Updates in
Hysteroscopy

Updates in
Hysteroscopy

Editors

Sushma Deshmukh MD DGO
Director
Central India Test Tube Baby Center
Head
Department of Obstetrics and Gynecology
Getwell Multispecialty Hospital and Research Center
In-charge of Deshmukh Hospital
Nagpur, Maharashtra, India

Osama Shawki MD
Professor of Gynecologic Surgery
Department of Gynecology
Cairo University, School of Medicine
Editor, European Journal of Gynecologic Surgery
Faculty Professor, Giessen School of Endoscopy, Germany
Board Member, International Society Gynecologic Endoscopy (ISGE)
Director of Ebtesama Center for Advanced Endoscopic Surgery
Director, Hysteroscopy Academy for Research and Training (HART)
Al Ebtesama Hospital, Heliopolis, Cairo, Egypt

Foreword
Luigi Montevecchi

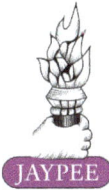

JAYPEE BROTHERS MEDICAL PUBLISHERS
The Health Sciences Publisher
New Delhi | London

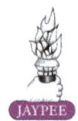
Jaypee Brothers Medical Publishers (P) Ltd

Headquarters
Jaypee Brothers Medical Publishers (P) Ltd
EMCA House, 23/23-B
Ansari Road, Daryaganj
New Delhi 110 002, India
Landline: +91-11-23272143, +91-11-23272703
+91-11-23282021, +91-11-23245672
Email: jaypee@jaypeebrothers.com

Corporate Office
Jaypee Brothers Medical Publishers (P) Ltd
4838/24, Ansari Road, Daryaganj
New Delhi 110 002, India
Phone: +91-11-43574357
Fax: +91-11-43574314
Email: jaypee@jaypeebrothers.com

Overseas Office
JP Medical Ltd
83 Victoria Street, London
SW1H 0HW (UK)
Phone: +44 20 3170 8910
Fax: +44 (0)20 3008 6180
Email: info@jpmedpub.com

Website: www.jaypeebrothers.com
Website: www.jaypeedigital.com

© 2024, Jaypee Brothers Medical Publishers

The views and opinions expressed in this book are solely those of the original contributor(s)/author(s) and do not necessarily represent those of editor(s) or publisher of the book.

All rights reserved. No part of this publication may be reproduced, stored or transmitted in any form or by any means, electronic, mechanical, photocopying, recording or otherwise, without the prior permission in writing of the publishers.

All brand names and product names used in this book are trade names, service marks, trademarks or registered trademarks of their respective owners. The publisher is not associated with any product or vendor mentioned in this book.

Medical knowledge and practice change constantly. This book is designed to provide accurate, authoritative information about the subject matter in question. However, readers are advised to check the most current information available on procedures included and check information from the manufacturer of each product to be administered, to verify the recommended dose, formula, method and duration of administration, adverse effects and contraindications. It is the responsibility of the practitioner to take all appropriate safety precautions. Neither the publisher nor the author(s)/editor(s) assume any liability for any injury and/or damage to persons or property arising from or related to use of material in this book.

This book is sold on the understanding that the publisher is not engaged in providing professional medical services. If such advice or services are required, the services of a competent medical professional should be sought.

Every effort has been made where necessary to contact holders of copyright to obtain permission to reproduce copyright material. If any have been inadvertently overlooked, the publisher will be pleased to make the necessary arrangements at the first opportunity.

Inquiries for bulk sales may be solicited at: jaypee@jaypeebrothers.com

Updates in Hysteroscopy

First Edition: **2024**

ISBN: 978-93-5696-745-8

Dedication

Dedicated to My Parents
Dr PR and Dr Sarojini Deshmukh
Who are constant source of inspiration for me
Enlightening my life and path
Supporting with Divine Touch

CONTRIBUTORS

Aditi Joshi Godbole
MBBS MS (Obs & Gyne) DNB (Obs & Gyne)
Shree Hospital
Kalyan, Maharashtra, India

Ashish Kale MD (Obs & Gyne) FICS MBBS
Consultant
Dr Ashish Kale's IVF Center
Pune, Maharashtra, India

Bernardo Portugal Lasmar MD
Professor of Gynecology
Maternal-Infant
Department of the Faculty of Medicine
of the Fluminense Federal University
UFF, Niterói, Rio de Janeiro, Brazil
Professor of Gynecology
at Estácio de Sá University (UNESA), Brazil
Responsible for Gynecological
Endoscopy at
Hospital Central Aristarcho Pessoa
HCAP-CBMERJ
Master in Gynecology from the
Fluminense Federal University, UFF

Carugno Jose MD
Medical Doctor
Department of Obstetrics, Gynecology
and Reproductive Sciences
Minimally Invasive Gynecology Division
University of Miami
Miller School of Medicine
Miami, Florida, USA

Giampietro Gubbini MD
Consultant
Madre Fortunata Toniolo Hospital
Bologna, Italy

José Luís Metello MD
Medical Doctor
Department of Gynecology and
Hysteroscopy
Hospital Garcia de Orta
Almada, Portugal

Jui Telang DGO
Consultant
Galaxy Care Hospital/Indira
Maternity Home
Pune, Maharashtra, India

Kalyan B Barmade
MBBS DNB DGO FCPS DFP
Managing Director
Barmade Hospital and Latur Fertility and
Endoscopy Center
Latur, Maharashtra, India

Luigi Montevecchi MD
Specialist in Obstetrics and Gynecology
Private Practice
Rome, Italy

Manisha K Barmade MBBS DGO
Consultant
Barmade Hospital and Latur Fertility and
Endoscopy Center
Latur, Maharashtra, India

Maria Chiara De Angelis MD PhD
Medical Doctor
Department of Public Health, School of
Medicine
University of Naples Federico II
Naples, Italy

Mario Franchini MD
Consultant
Demetra IVF Center-Vila Cherubini
Florence, Italy

Milind A Telang MD DGO DNB
Endoscopic Surgeon and IVF
Consultant
Galaxy Care Hospital/Indira Maternity
Home
Pune, Maharashtra, India

Mykhailo V Medvediev MD PhD ScD
Professor
Department of Obstetrics and
Gynecology
Dnipro State Medical University
Dnipro, Ukraine

Nagendra Sardeshpande
DNB FCPS DGO DFP MBBS
Consultant, Gynecologic Endoscopic
Surgeon
Bombay Hospital Institute of Medical
Sciences
Mumbai, Maharashtra, India

Nitin Shah
MS (Obs & Gyne) DNB (Obs & Gyne) FCPS
(General Surgery) DGO
Vardaan Multispecialty
Mumbai, Maharashtra, India

Osama Shawki MD
Professor of Gynecologic Surgery
Department of Gynecology
Cairo University, School of Medicine
Editor, European Journal of Gynecologic
Surgery
Faculty Professor, Giessen School of
Endoscopy, Germany
Board Member, International Society
Gynecologic Endoscopy (ISGE)
Director of Ebtesama Center for
Advanced Endoscopic Surgery
Director, Hysteroscopy Academy for
Research and Training (HART)
Al Ebtesama Hospital
Heliopolis, Cairo, Egypt

Pandit Palaskar
MBBS MD DNBE DFP MNAMS Diploma
Endoscopic Surgery (Australia)
Consultant
Endoworld Hospital
Aurangabad, Maharashtra, India

Pankaj Mate MD DGO FMIS FICG
Consultant, Laparoscopic Gynecologist
Galaxy Care Multispecialty Hospital
Pvt Ltd
Pune, Maharashtra, India
Advanced Care in Laparoscopic
Surgery

Paolo Casadio MD
Consultant
Division of Gynecology and
Human Reproduction Physiopathology
IRCCS Azienda Ospedaliero-Universitaria
di Bologna
Bologna, Italy

Patrícia Nazaré MD
Medical Doctor
Department of Gynecology and
Hysteroscopy Hospital Garcia de Orta
Almada, Portugal

Rajesh Gajbhiye MBBS MD
Consultant, Laparoscopic Surgeon
Department of Obstetrician and
Gynecologist
Mauli Women's Hospital
Nagpur, Maharashtra, India

Ricardo Bassil Lasmar MD PhD
Professor of Gynecology
Department of Surgery and Specialized
Faculty of Medicine
Universidade Federal Fluminense, UFF,
Niterói, Rio de Janeiro, Brazil
Member of National Specialized
Commission on Gynecological
Endoscopy of the FEBRASGO
Member of the Brazilian College of
Surgeons

S Krishnakumar
MBBS MD (Midwifery & Gynecology)
Chief Consultant
JK Women Hospital, Dombivali
Consultant at Fortis Hospital
Immediate Past President of IAGE

Sandeep Nikhade MD
Consultant
Lifesprings Hospital
Nagpur, Maharashtra, India

Sergio Haimovich MD PhD
Medical Doctor
Department of Obstetrics and Gynecology
Laniado University Hospital
Netanya
Israel and Adelson School of Medicine
Ariel University, Ariel, Israel

Sergio Haimovich MD PhD
Professor and Head
Hysteroscopy Unit
Del Mar University Hospital
Barcelona, Spain

Shashikant Raghuwanshi
MBBS MS (Obs & Gyne) FMIS
Consultant
Raghuwanshi Hospital and Research
Center, Ramdspeth
Nagpur, Maharashtra, India

Shrutika O Makde
MS (Obs & Gyne) DNB (Obs & Gyne) ICOG
Infertility Fellow
Consultant
Department of Obstetrics and
Gynecology
Lokmanya Tilak Municipal General
Hospital and Medical College
Mumbai, Maharashtra, India

Sushma Deshmukh MD DGO
Director
Central India Test Tube Baby Center
Head
Department of Obstetrics and
Gynecology
Getwell Multispecialty Hospital and
Research Center
In-charge of Deshmukh Hospital
Nagpur, Maharashtra, India

Tanvir Singh MBBS MS (Obs & Gyne)
Consultant
Tanvir Hospital
Hyderabad, Telangana, India

FOREWORD

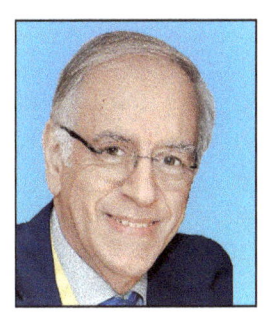

The history of hysteroscopy dates back to the 19th century. In fact, it was the Italian Pantaleoni who performed the first hysteroscopy in 1869 and completed it successfully.

Since then, there have been countless technological innovations, and from lighting techniques to distension media, from the creation of new instruments to the most varied indications, hysteroscopy has undergone a transformation that was unthinkable only 40 years ago.

This manual, edited by Sushma Deshmukh and Osama Shawki, was created to fill an information gap: its structure, of a predominantly practical nature, aims to facilitate the learning of some diagnostic and surgical hysteroscopy techniques, and to provide an update on the most recent applications of the branch.

The basic requirements and equipment for carrying out an outpatient hysteroscopy are analyzed (Chapters 1, 2, 3 and 4), the pathologies that can be addressed with the hysteroscopic technique are investigated, from the most frequent to the most innovative ones (Chapters 5-17), and suggested measures for preventing complications, using simple practical tips (Chapters 18 and 19).

Overall, this update manual will satisfy those who want practical answers to everyday questions, without having to spend excessive time delving into each individual topic.

Once you have obtained the answers to your doubts or curiosities, nothing prevents you from dedicating the remaining time to consulting the individual bibliographic entries, to broaden your hysteroscopic culture.

Luigi Montevecchi MD
Specialist in Obstetrics and Gynecology
Private Practice
Rome, Italy

PREFACE

Hysteroscopy is gaining importance day by day and has become one of the top modalities of evaluation, diagnosis as well as for treatment. Hysteroscope is one of the important wonder instruments that each and every gynecologist must have in their basket. But the beauty of hysteroscope is that it can be used in office settings without anesthesia as investigating modality and blessed with treating capacity in the same settings, i.e., See and Treat.

I have written three books on hysteroscopy. Why need of fourth book? My every book is different. This time I have planned manual with practical tips. Due to advancement in technology, every year many new upcoming technologies, new guidelines are entering in Hysteroscopy world. And the beginners and hysteron-lovers must know it. So, I have designed the book in a different way. We are having very practical difficulties while carrying out hysteroscopic surgeries. So, we need a quick reference book. So, this manual is a ready reckoner in true sense. To arrange the hysteroscopy set up from the beginning with proper selection of equipments is very important. Office hysteroscopy one needs to learn as it requires specific instruments and precise movements. Intrauterine surgeries like Septum, Polyp, Myoma, Retained products of conception, Intrauterine adhesions are becoming regular and we need to learn the concepts. Tuberculosis is affecting endometrium and affecting gestosis in India and developing countries. Hysteroscopy is not easy surgery and we need to understand the limitations and precautions to avoid the complications. And lastly, we must respect the Mother Womb and work for save uterus.

Sushma Deshmukh

ACKNOWLEDGMENTS

To design a masterpiece and execute with exceptional mind body work is very much satisfying. But behind this craftsmanship a team of helping hands is always there. For them it is a simple work, but for us it is a blessing. After a wonderful journey of three books in Hysteroscopy, we decided to plan Hysteroscopy manual which will be easy to refer for day-to-day practice. And it is a good opportunity for us to release this manual in Nagpur Hysteroscopy Carnival-III in collaboration with Indian Association of Gynecological Endoscopists with Nagpur Obstetric and Gynecological Society. And we are really thankful to all associations.

Our heartfelt thanks to M/s Jaypee Brothers Medical Publishers (P) Ltd, New Delhi, India for genesis of this book. It has compelled us to work hard putting new ideas to give justice to their confidence in us. Special thanks to Shri Jitendar P Vij (Group Chairman) who always says "Yes" to all academic work. Thanks to Mr Ankit Vij (Managing Director), Ms Chetna Malhotra (Senior Director—Professional Publishing, Marketing, and Business Development), Ms Manpreet Kaur (Development Editor), and Ms Kritika Dua (Senior Commissioning Editor), and all loving Jaypee family for bringing this book for readers.

Our many national and international faculties really took great pains to write their practical views in their chapters. Thanks to all.

In this academic journey, our families supported us by sparing their quality time and encouraging us always. We are thankful to Almighty God who is always there to guide us.

Me and My Hysteroscope

I know, My Hysteroscope
In Obs-Gyne is having lot of scope
In the cavity when we enter,
Me and My Hysteroscope
Always talk together
Is this normal endometrium?
Or that looks like a septum?
I can deal with scissors
Occasionally mono-Bipolar
Locate surprise polyp
Can be managed with scissors/forceps
Myoma, Isthmocele, Adhesion
Retained products of conception
Proximal tubal occlusion
Any abnormal bleeding
BOH or Infertility
And the list is unending.....
For rewarding results just try-
In all phases of life
In can make comfortable life!

CONTENTS

1. **Introduction and Basic Requirements for Hysteroscopy** 1
   Sushma Deshmukh

2. **Instruments for Hysteroscopy** 5
   Nagendra Sardeshpande

3. **Distension Media, Pressure System, and Electrosurgical Unit in Hysteroscopy** 13
   Shashikant Raghuwanshi, Rajesh Gajbhiye, Sandeep Nikhade

4. **Office Hysteroscopy** 19
   Nitin Shah, Aditi Joshi Godbole

5. **Endometrial Polyp: How to Deal with it?** 24
   Sergio Haimovich, Tanvir Singh

6. **Septum and Management Plan** 29
   Tanvir Singh

7. **Mullerian Anomalies Other than Septum: Role of Hysteroscopy** 35
   Ashish Kale

8. **Intrauterine Adhesions: Systematic Approach** 45
   S Krishnakumar, Shrutika O Makde

9. **Submucous Myoma: Best Possible Ways** 53
   Ricardo Bassil Lasmar, Bernardo Portugal Lasmar

10. **Chronic Endometritis, Tuberculosis, and Hysteroscopy** 59
    Sushma Deshmukh

11. **Isthmocele: Smart Use of Hysteroscopy** 66
    Mario Franchini, Paolo Casadio, Giampietro Gubbini

12. **Proximal Tubal Cannulation, Making Simplified** 72
    Mykhailo V Medvediev

13. **Hysteroscopy in Retained Products of Conception** 76
    Milind A Telang, Jui Telang

14. **Misplaced Foreign Bodies in the Uterine Cavity** 78
    Pankaj Mate

15. **Cervix Under Microscope** 84
    Luigi Montevecchi

16. **Hysteroscopy in Postmenopausal Bleeding** 92
    Kalyan B Barmade, Pandit Palaskar, Manisha K Barmade

17. **Expanded Scope of Hysteroscopy: Embryoscopy, Cesarean Section Scar Ectopic Pregnancy, Tubal Sterilization** 95
    Carugno Jose, Maria Chiara De Angelis, Sergio Haimovich

18. **Anticipating, Preventing, and Managing Complications in Hysteroscopy** 101
    Patrícia Nazaré, José Luís Metello

19. **Practical Tips in Operative Hysteroscopy** 106
    Osama Shawki

Index *111*

Introduction and Basic Requirements for Hysteroscopy

Chapter 1

Sushma Deshmukh

The evolution of hysteroscopy was on unusual score.
It has followed an atypical career in medical folklore.
Initially there were the case reports and biased opinions.
Then a brief case series but a very long gestation.
Though this invention is a worldly creation.
It developed through delayed milestones.
It almost took a century for hysteroscopy to gain importance.
Taken care by the concerned one, accepting critics and honors.
Resulting in an extraordinary outcome!

INTRODUCTION

Hysteroscopy is an endo ART (admirable rewarding technology). It has pioneered the process of endoscopic viewing of uterine cavity with less invasive form of treatment. Step-by-step in the present scenario hysteroscopy ranks as one the topmost modalities.

PHILOSOPHY OF UTERUS AND HYSTEROSCOPE

- (Womb) "hustera", i.e., womb a Latin word. The term "hysteroscopy" is derived from the fusion of two ancient Greek words "histeros" (uterus) and "scopeo" (to see).
- Uterus is the most dynamic and adjustable organ in mammals. In human, it is in full form from menarche to menopause. Under the influence of sex hormones, the uterus undergoes various changes from a smaller prepubertal size to normal adult size and in expansion phase during pregnancy.
- To view the "hystera" through hysteroscopy is like learning the philosophy of hystera, i.e., uterus. The hysteroscope is also designed in a delicate way to adjust the curves of uterus, to occupy space in the uterus without disturbing its anatomy and physiology

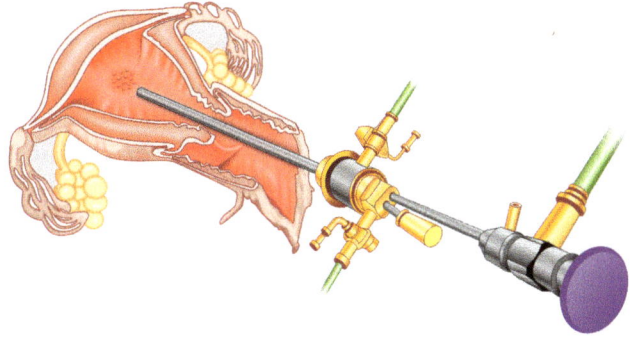

Fig. 1: Uterus and hysteroscope.

(Fig. 1). That is why today most of the hysteroscopic procedures do not need anesthesia.

How to begin with hysteroscopy?
- *Change the mindset:* From impossible to I am possible
- Gather all information
- Indications for hysteroscopy
- Selection of patient should be proper
- Set up of hysteroscopy unit
- Counseling before office hysteroscopy (OH)

Change the Mindset

From impossible to I am possible with determination, motivation, and inspiration. One should be ready for up gradation.

Remember that though hysteroscopy appears simple, it is not like that.

Learn that there is only one entry point. All operating instruments pass through the same entry point.
- No luxury of assistants
- No luxury of putting many instruments
- Cannot use another hand for holding operative instrument with any tissue
- Time limit because of chances of fluid overload
- Totally depends on good visualization

Gather All Information about Hysteroscopy

Start attending workshops, training and visit the places to get hands on training which will also help in organizing the proper room, instruments, and equipments.

Indications for Hysteroscopy

- *Evaluation of abnormal uterine bleeding:* About 25–30% of patients are of abnormal polyps, submucous fibroids. Plain D and C misses the pathology in 30% of patients. Hysteroscopy-directed biopsy is definitely superior to blind D and C/endometrial biopsy.
- *Evaluation of infertility:* Mullerian anomalies, adhesions, polyps, submucous fibroid, and endometrial pattern
- Evaluation in recurrent pregnancy loss, especially uterine septum
- Misplaced or lost intrauterine contraceptive device
- Hysteroscopic sterilization
- Prior to in vitro fertilization (IVF) cycle
- Endometrial cancer
- *Obstetrics:* Retained products of conception (RPOC), scar ectopic pregnancy, isthmocele, and many more indications.

Selection of Patient

- Always plan hysteroscopy postmenstrually except suspected tuberculosis
- Start with simple cases, multiparous
- Evaluate with transvaginal sonography (TVS) properly to avoid sudden surprises
- *Proper fitness:* In high risk patients, there is advantage of OH as no anesthesia is required

Many studies showed that nulliparity, cervical pathology, and procedures over 2 minutes in length were correlated with severe pain in OH.

So, the newcomers can begin initially with diagnostic hysteroscopy in multiparous patients without cervical pathology to allow for building confidence to progress to operative hysteroscopy.

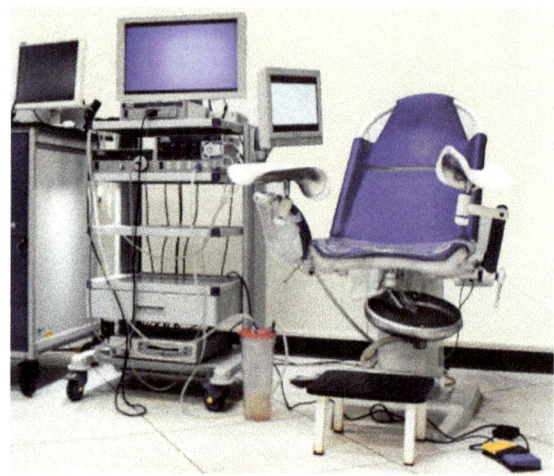

Fig. 2: Mobile cart with chair.

Set up of Hysteroscopy Unit

To begin with, one should have basic knowledge of essential instruments on the mobile cart and trolley.

The three important things in outpatient/OT hysteroscopy clinics are:
1. Good quality equipments and optics
2. Comfort of patient and surgeon
3. Adequately trained, skilled assistants.

Good Quality Equipments and Optics

i. Nicely furnished room with hydraulic table/chair with comfortable stirrups.
ii. Mobile cart containing monitor, camera unit with recording system, xenon light source with fiber optic cable, pressure pump like endomat and electrosurgical unit on the left side of surgeon **(Fig. 2)**.
   - *Distension media:* Nowadays, normal saline is used as distension media. And hystero-pump endomat, which allows monitoring of irrigation and suction pressure, controls flow rate or medex pressure bags. Generally we require very minimal pressure of 40–50 mm and we can increase up to 70–80 mm according to case.
   - *Camera system:* One should have good camera system if possible high-definition camera system for better resolution
   - *Light source and light cable:* Various light sources are available like Halogen, LED, and Xenon. It is preferable to use Xenon.

- *Recording system:* One should remember that each and every video should be recorded
- *Electrosurgical unit and electrodes:* When we are using normal saline as a distension media then bipolar cautery is used when needed. In monopolar current, glycine is used.

iii. *Instrument trolleys:*
   a. This is the trolley containing basic instruments of OH, i.e., see and treat
      - 2.9 mm 30 degree Bettocchi's operative office hysteroscope with continuous flow operative channel
      - 4.5 mm inner sheath and 5 mm outer sheath
      - 5 French scissors, forceps (grasping, biopsy) for removal of polyp, adhesions and for biopsy purpose.

      Even it is used for dilatation, negotiation, of internal/external ostium to proceed ahead.
   b. Instruments on another trolley like Sponge holder with gauze pieces and antiseptic solution speculum, vulsellum/tenaculum, endometrial biopsy cannula, etc.
   c. *Electrical instruments:*
      - Bipolar needle electrode, which can be used in 2.9 mm hysteroscope
      - *Resectoscope:* The resectoscope consists of a classic endoscope, with diameters ranging between 2.9 and 4 mm—preferably with a 30 viewing angle to keep the electrode within the field of view.

      It is combined with a cutting loop operated by a passive spring mechanism and two sheaths for continuous irrigation and suction of the distension medium. Apart from the cutting loop, other instruments such as Collin's knife and a variety of vaporizing or coagulating electrodes can be used with the working element of the resectoscope.

      All these instruments are available from 14-Fr to the 26-Fr resectoscope.
   d. *Proper placement in OT:* It is very important that all the things to be properly placed for hysteroscopy. Mobile cart on left side, trolley on right side, monitor on left side if possible another camera at front side of surgeon **(Fig. 3)**.

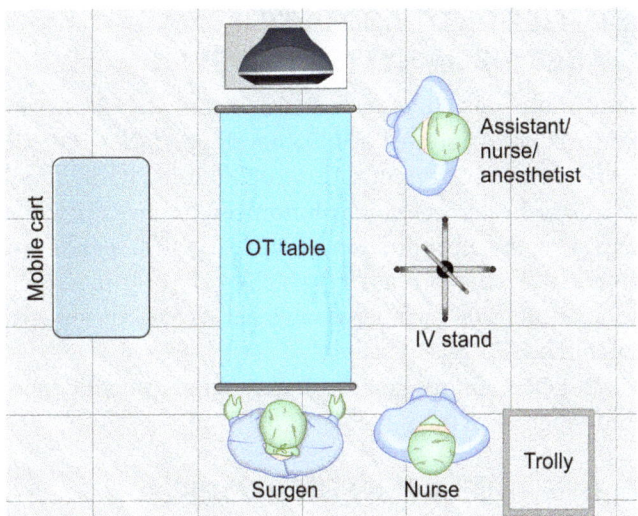

Fig. 3: Placement in OT.

Comfort of Patient and Surgeon

- *Position of the patient:*
  - One should always remember that correct lithotomy position is necessary, i.e., with legs apart supported in leg rests with the buttocks at the edge of the table or few cms extending beyond the table.
  - Ask patient to relax and back should be flat to avoid postoperative back strain.
  - Comfortable leg rests and joint in the leg should not be flexed over 60° to avoid femoral nerve compression (associated with extreme flexion, abduction and lateral rotation of hip).
- *Position of the surgeon:*
  - The surgeon should be comfortable and need to sit between the patient's leg and the eye level of the patient and surgeon should match.
  - According to angle of uterus, chair should be adjusted. In acutely anteverted uterus, the surgeon's chair should be at lower level and in acutely retroverted at a higher level.
  - Some surgeons recommend standing position as the movements will be at wrist and elbow level. In this case, the camera and the telescope should be at or just below the lower border of umbilicus.
  - In a sitting position, the movements will be at wrist elbow and shoulder level giving more strain. In this case, whole system should be at few inches above the level of umbilicus.

Counseling before Office Hysteroscopy

Proper counseling of the patient is very important especially in OH. Patient should understand the procedure and should have confidence with the surgeon as well as the office procedure.

OFFICE OR OT AND UNDER ANESTHESIA HYSTEROSCOPY

The whole world is now moving toward OH. Professor Bettocchi and Selvaggi in 1995 developed a NO-TOUCH VAGINOSCOPY technique which along with small diameter hysteroscope revolutionized the hysteroscopy and also the introduction of VERSAPOINT generator (under water bipolar cautery) which can be used in normal saline distension media leads to what is called as modern operative OH.

But OH requires great patience, patient's confidence, and expertise of the surgeon.

TIPS AND TRICKS PERFORMING OFFICE HYSTEROSCOPY

- Always select proper patient for proper indication and rule out contraindication.
- Patient and surgeon positioning should be perfect.
- Proper training of nurse involved in the procedure with respect to procedure instrumentation
- Procedure to be performed in the immediate postmenstrual phase
- *Preprocedure*: Analgesics, atropine misoprostol can be used in OH as per choice of surgeon. Usually, it is not needed.
- Vaginal preparation not usually required. Antibiotics can be given.
- Verbal anesthesia while performing the procedure
- Routine local anesthesia—blocks not required if miniature hysteroscopes are used. But can be used in certain cases—menopausal myomectomy in OH.
- Use normal saline as distension media of room temperature easily convertible from diagnostic to operative with bipolar system, less complications
- Always work with low pressure. Avoid high pressure and let saline (fluid) open up the path.
- Hold the labia, guide scope to cervix with finger, stabilize the uterus with the fundal pressure.
- Learn proper technique while negotiating the internal os and examining the uterine cavity.
- Decrease the pressure while coming out of the uterine cavity
- Patient's consideration is the priority, comfort of patient
- Gentle and precise movements of the surgeon
- Distraction of patient with conversation, music, and prayer
- No touch, no pressure over myometrium
- Be instrument friendly
- Work with affectionate heart, be compassionate.

CONCLUSION

- Office hysteroscopy is a safe and effective option for diagnosis and management of intrauterine pathology.
- Primary uses of hysteroscopy include diagnosis of abnormal uterine bleeding and treating endometrial polyps, uterine septa, retained products of pregnancy, and adhesions.
- Upgradation requires proper training and instruments set up.
- Equipment selection should be based on the types of procedures planned for the office/OT setting.
- Appropriate patient selection is the most important component for both patient and physician comfort when starting a hysteroscopy program.

Success of hysteroscopic procedures depends upon good hysteroscopy unit, surgeon, dedication, and learning updates.

So in hysteroscopy, if you learn with dedication then the further steps are: beginning–learning–motivation–upgradation–disclosing mystery–revealing magic and one will start learning and loving hysteroscopy again and again.

Instruments for Hysteroscopy

Chapter 2

Nagendra Sardeshpande

INTRODUCTION

Hysteroscopy: A Window into the Uterine World.

Hysteroscopy is a procedure that involves direct visual inspection of cervical canal and uterine cavity.

Instrumentation is at the heart of hysteroscopy, as it equips healthcare providers with the necessary tools to navigate and visualize the uterine cavity. In this chapter, we delve into the world of hysteroscopic instrumentation, exploring the key components that make this procedure both safe and effective.[1]

INSTRUMENTS

Endoscope

It is a rigid telescope that has three parts: (1) The eyepiece, (2) the barrel, and (3) the objective lens. Focal length and angle of distal tip are important for visualization.

Angle options include 0, 12, 15, 30, and 70. A 0° hysteroscope provides a panoramic view while an angled one might improve the view of ostia in an abnormally shaped uterus.

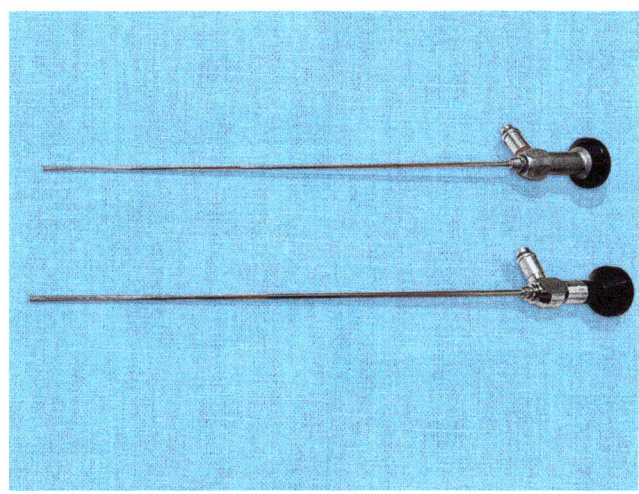

Fig. 1: The 4-mm and 2.9-mm hysteroscopes.

There are three types of endoscopes **(Fig. 1)**.

1. *Rigid hysteroscope (Hopkins hysteroscope):* The standard used rigid hysteroscope is 4 mm with a 5-mm diagnostic sheath. This scope provides a very good image. It is available with varying directions of view: 0, 12, or 30°. Normally, a 30° scope is used for diagnosis while a 12° scope is used for operative work such as endometrial resection. However, a 30° scope can also be used for resection.

    In case of operative procedures, the 4-mm scope needs to be combined with an operative sheath with a diameter of 70–8.5 mm, necessitating anesthesia and cervical dilatation.

2. *The mini rigid 2.9-mm/1.9-mm office hysteroscope:* In order to overcome the shortcomings of a standard 4-mm scope, there have evolved two systems that can be effectively utilized for diagnostic and operative hysteroscopy, either in an outpatient office setting or an inpatient hospital setting.

    With these systems, it is possible to perform operative procedures such as polypectomy (polyps <4 cm diameter), adhesiolysis, tubal cannulations, and myomectomies (myomas <2 cm) in an office setting.

    The standard Bettocchi hysteroscope (Karl Storz): This hysteroscope with Hopkins based rods lens system is a miniature version of the famous Hamou-2 microhysteroscope. The scope has an external diameter of 2.9 mm. It can be used as a panoramic hysteroscope (1×) as well as a micro contact hysteroscope (80×). The scope is also available without the microhysteroscopic attachment (commonly used by the author). For diagnostic purposes, it can be used with a single flow outer sheath of 3.6 mm or a continuous flow outer sheath of 4.4 mm. In case of operative hysteroscopy, it can be combined with a continuous flow operative sheath of 3.9 mm × 5.9 mm (average diameter 5 mm). This sheath has an operative channel to accommodate 5 French instruments to pass through for operative purpose.[2]

The modified Bettocchi: This is a new version with a 1.9-mm diameter optic along with corresponding decreased diameters of diagnostic and operative sheath.

The semi-rigid Versascope system (Johnson and Johnson—Gynecare division) **(Fig. 2)**: The Versascope is a flexible telescope made up of a set of 50,000 fused optical fibers, providing a 0° field of vision with an outer panoramic angle view of 75°. The scope has an external diameter of 1.8 mm and length of 28 cm. The density and optical quality of the image system produces an image, which is similar to the conventional rod lens panoramic hysteroscope. Unlike the rigid scopes, the Versascope has got a disposable sheath. It is used with a continuous flow diagnostic cum operative sheath, which has an outer diameter of 3.5 mm and a distal curvature of 10°. A proximal collar is provided. This can be rotated through 360°. This allows manipulation of the scope for full peripheral viewing, without disturbing the instrument position. The operative channel has an expandable instrument channel which can easily accommodate instruments till 7 French in diameter. This operative channel also simultaneously functions as an independent outflow port for continuous flow during the procedure. The hysteroscope comes with a fiberoptic cable.

The Versascope is no longer available.

3. *Flexible hysteroscope* **(Figs. 3A and B)**: It is 1.2-mm fiberoptic hysteroscope with soft flexible front section and rigid in middle. Newer devices with integrated fiberoptic hysteroscope and diagnostic cum operative sheath are available (Endosee) with an inbuilt light source and a small handheld size monitor integrated with the viewing lens of the hysteroscope. This is a disposable system which can be used in an outpatient based office hysteroscopy and is capable of performing

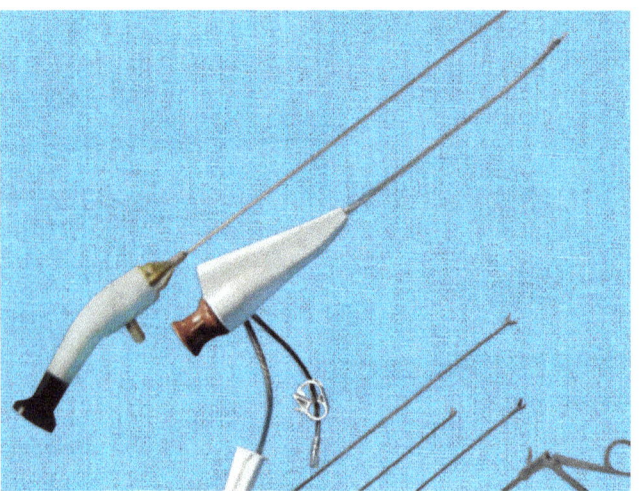

Fig. 2: The Versascope.

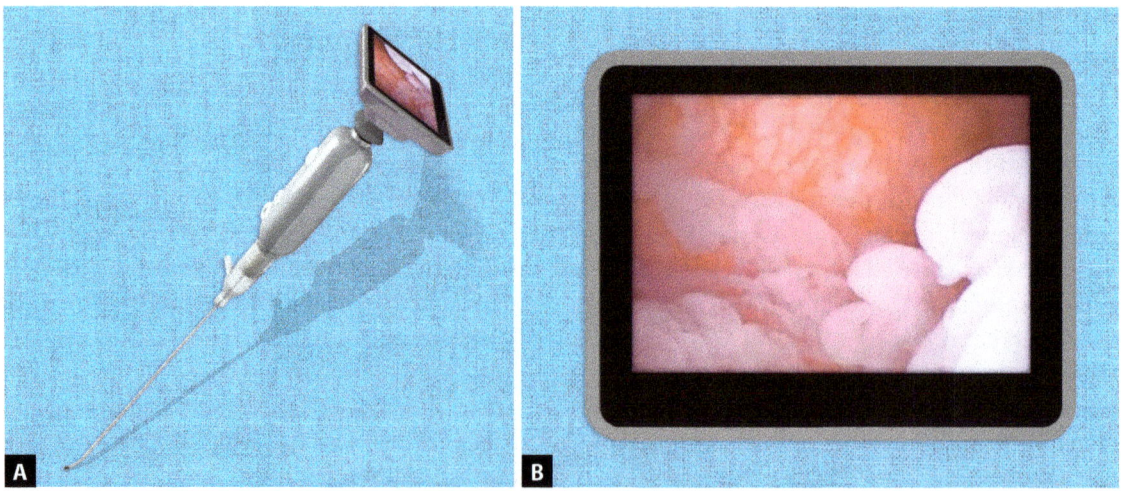

Figs. 3A and B: (A) The EndoSee flexible integrated disposable office hysteroscopy system; (B) Image seen on EndoSee monitor.

minor operative procedures such as polypectomy, metroplasty, and removal of foreign bodies.

Advantages:
- Can be easily passed into the uterine cavity without dilatation[3]
- Fine operative procedures such as embryo transfer
- Diagnostic and operative procedures in irregular shape uterus

Disadvantages:
- Very fragile and generates a small image
- Extremely costly and very delicate

4. *Microhysteroscope:* It is combination of panoramic hysteroscopy, contrast hysteroscopy, and microscopy which is a high-powered microscope and needs contact of light and hysteroscope to the mucous membrane (endometrium). It can be used to perform retrograde salpingoscopy before tuboplasty.[4,5]

Sheaths

Telescope has a sheath which encases it leaving 1 mm gap between inner wall and telescope for transfer of distension media. It fits by a watertight seal lock.

Diameter depends on the diameter of telescope used.[6]

There are two types of sheaths:
1. *Diagnostic sheaths (Fig. 4):* About 4–5 mm in diameter to allow passage of telescope and distension media.
2. *Operative sheaths (Figs. 5A to C):* Larger diameter (7–10 mm) to allow insertion of telescope, distension media, and operative devices.

Sheath for 2.9-mm Bettocchi scope:
- Single flow 36-mm diagnostic sheath
- Continuous flow 3.6-mm inner sheath along with 4.4-mm outer sheath for diagnostic hysteroscopy
- Single flow 4.3-mm operating sheath which has got a channel for introducing 2-mm operating instruments
- Continuous flow 4.3-mm inner sheath along with 5-mm outer sheath for diagnostic as well as all operative procedures. This combination is the best to have.
- Recently, there is a new smaller diameter resectoscope sheaths with inner and outer cannels along with

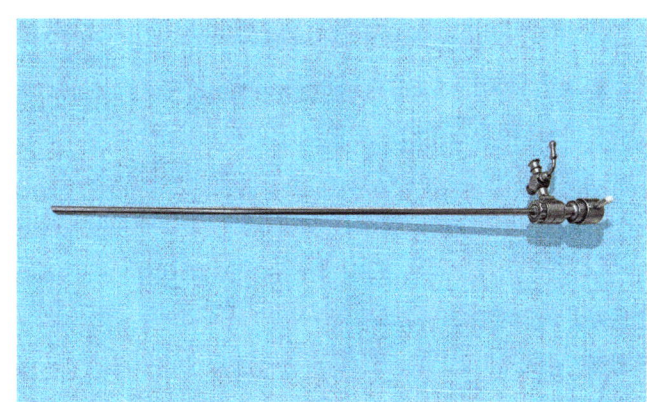

Fig. 4: The diagnostic sheath.

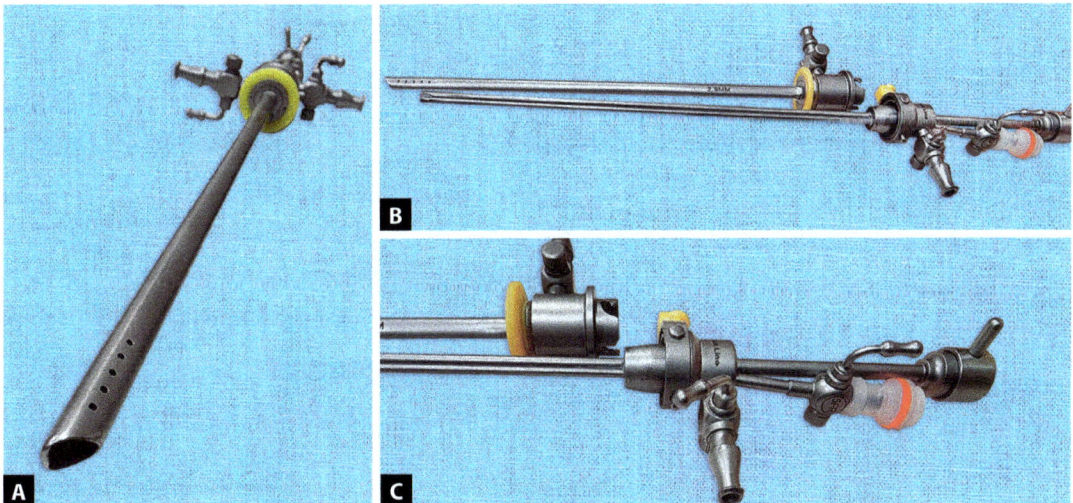

Figs. 5A to C: (A) The assembled operating sheath; (B) The outer and inner channels of the operating sheath; (C) The inner channel allows passage of the operating instruments and the hysteroscopy irrigation fluid whereas the outer channel allows outflow of fluid along with debris.

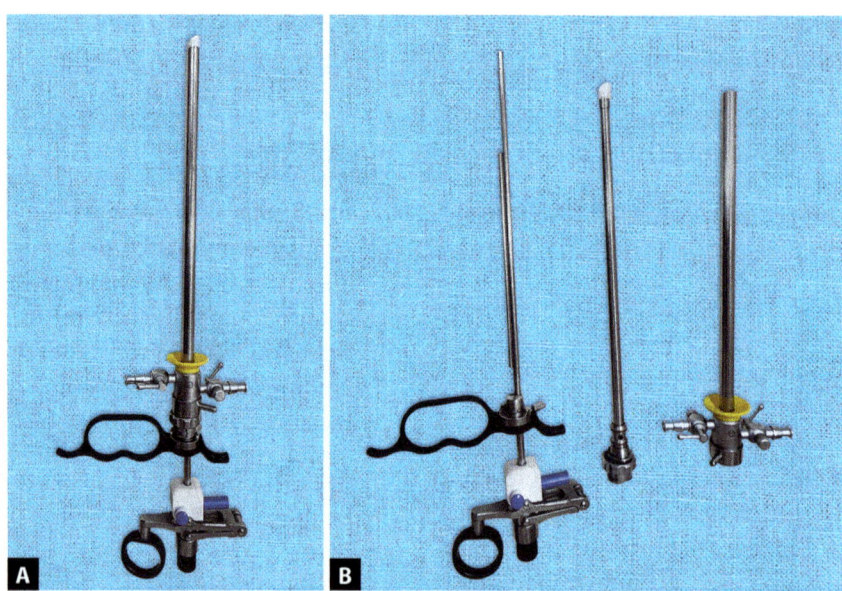

Figs. 6A and B: (A) The assembled resectoscope; (B) The various parts of the resectoscope from right to left: the outer sheath, the inner sheath, and the working element.

smaller diameter electrodes (loop, ball, cylinder, and knife) which can be used with the 2.9-mm Bettocchi scope.

Sheaths for the 4-mm standard hysteroscope:
- Single flow sheath for diagnosis
- Continuous flow with inner and outer sheath for diagnosis
- Continuous flow inner and outer sheath for operative purpose along with operative channel.

Resectoscope (Figs. 6A and B): Resectoscope is a specialized electrosurgical (monopolar or bipolar endoscope) which consists of an inner sheath and an outer sheath. The inner sheath has a common channel for the telescope, fluid medium, and electrode, while the outer sheath is for fluid return. The electrode is fitted to a trigger device which pushes the electrode beyond the sheath and then pulls it back within the sheath.

The operating tools have four basic electrodes:
1. A cutting loop
2. Ball electrode
3. Button
4. Angulated needle

Types:
- Standard 26-mm resectoscope with inner sheath, outer sheath, working element, and electrodes for using unipolar current
- Standard 26-mm resectoscope (Gynecare Johnson) with inner sheath, outer sheath, working element, and bipolar electrodes to be used with Versapoint bipolar current. It is important to note that this sheath has to be used with standard 2.9-mm or 4-mm Hopkins rigid hysteroscope. It cannot be combined with the Versascope.

Light Cables
- Standard fiberoptic cable to be used with Hopkins endoscopes and cold light source or xenon light source. The cable is normally 5 mm in diameter and 180 cm in length.
- Special fused fiber light cable to be used with Versascope. This cable can be attached to any type of light source with special adaptors.

Light Source
There are various light sources, which one can use for illumination:
- *Halogen:* This 150–250 watts cold light source is sufficient for vision. However, it tends to give of a reddish tinge to the image.
- *Xenon:* A 175 watts xenon light source provides an outstanding illumination and enables a good depth of field. Although the light is extremely hot at its source, most of the heat gets dissipated along the length of the

fiberoptic cable. Despite this, a significant amount of heat can be generated at the distal tip. This can cause thermal injury to the patient or burn paper drapes or clothing with prolonged contact. Hence, one should keep the intensity of the light as less as possible.

Camera

A single chip endoscopic camera is sufficient for diagnostic and minor operative work. A three chip camera will not be of additional help, unless it has additional filters to eliminate the pixelation and digitalization of the image.

The technical criteria of a good camera are:
- *Good resolution:* Based on the number of lines or pixels
- *High sensitivity:* Based on the lux
- High quality of video output images
- Good signal to noise ratio
- Easy sterilization system

Recording devices:
- Video
- Digital recording on CD/DVD

Monitors:
- Liquid crystal display (LCD) monitors
- Flat screen computers
- Flat screen televisions

Distension Media

Having a thick musculature, a minimum of 40 mm Hg pressure is needed to distend the uterine cavity. A pressure of 70 mm Hg is needed to propel the medium through fallopian tubes and peritoneal cavity for dye testing.

Types of distension media:
- *Gas:* Carbon dioxide
- *Liquid:*
  - High viscosity: Dextran 32%, Hyskon
  - Low viscosity:
    - Iso-osmolar (electrolyte):
      - Normal saline 0.9% (285 mOsm)
      - Ringers lactate (279 mOsm)
      - Nonelectrolyte mannitol 5% (274 mOsm)
    - Hypo-osmolar (nonelectrolyte):
      - Glycine 1.5% (200 mOsm)
      - Sorbitol 3% (165 mOsm)
      - Dextrose 5%

Liquid media: Most hospitals in India and in world use liquid media. The type of liquid media used are:

- *Normal saline (0.9%):* Sodium chloride is safest of all hysteroscopic media. A 3-liter (L) bottle is used for continuous infusion through dual channel operating sheath for constant flow rate in uterine cavity.

  It is cheap and easily available.

  However, it is not suitable for monopolar electrosurgery but is suitable for mechanical devices, bipolar cautery, and YAG and KTP laser. Fluid deficit (fluid given—retained fluid) of >1.0 L is indication of suspension of procedure to avoid complications of fluid overload.

- *Glycine (1.5%):* It was used in transurethral resection of prostate and is adopted by gynecologists. It is suitable for monopolar cautery and for electrosurgical devices like resectoscope.

Disadvantages:
- Being hypo-osmolar a fluid deficit should not be >750 mL
- It can cause hyponatremia and hypo-osmolarity and even deaths have been reported.
- It can be metabolized to ammonia and cause neurological damage.

Mechanical Operating System

Systems commonly used to control flow rate and irrigation pressure are:
- *Gravity fall of liquid:* The bag is suspended at a suitable height (90–100 cm from the patient's perineum is sufficient to obtain an irrigation pressure of approximately 70 mm Hg).
- *Pressure cuff* **(Fig. 7)***:* These are devices similar to sphygmomanometers which apply pressure around the bag. The pressure is obtained by inflating the pressure cuff, and must be kept at around 80 mm Hg by an assistant.
- *Electronic suction and irrigation pump* **(Fig. 8)***:* Automatic control of the suction and irrigation parameters is of paramount importance as hysteroscopic surgery continuously requires clear vision of the operating field, and constant distention of the uterine cavity.

Such units are commonly operated using three set values: (1) Flow rate approximately 200 mL/min, (2) irrigation pressure of 75 mm Hg, and (3) suction pressure of 0.25 bar, simply by readjusting the set values of flow rate and irrigation pressure, the "HAMOU ENDOMAT" can be used both for hysteroscopy and laparoscopy.

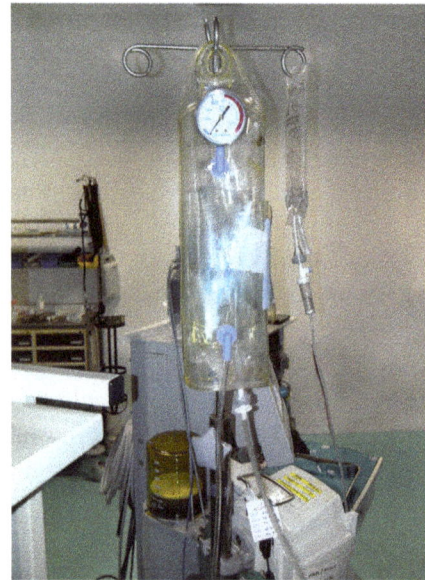

Fig. 7: Irrigation bag.

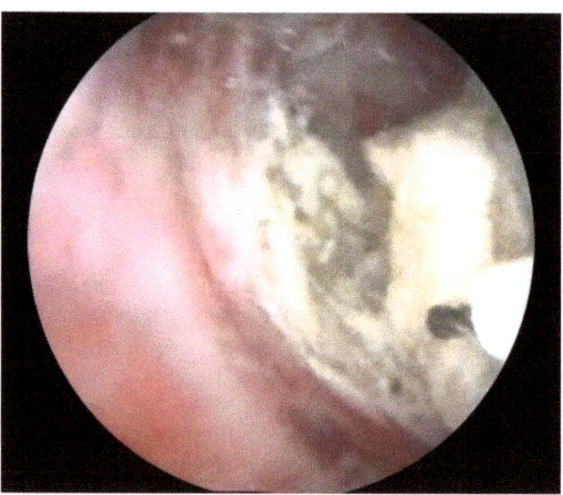

Fig. 9: Twizzle electrode.

2. Ball electrode
3. Spring electrode

These are used in combination with ionic distention media such as saline.

- *Unipolar resectoscope electrodes:* These are of four types **(Figs. 10A to D)**:
  1. Loop
  2. Rollerball
  3. Cylinder
  4. Calvins knife

  These have to be used in combination with monopolar cautery and glycine.
- *Bipolar Versapoint resectoscope electrodes:* These have to be used in combination with Versapoint bipolar cautery and saline.

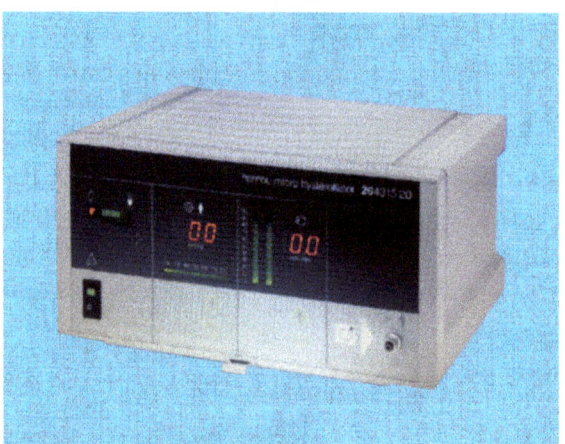

Fig. 8: Hysteromat.

Electrodes

- *Monopolar electrodes:* This 2-mm electrode uses monopolar energy and has to be used in combination with nonionic media such as glycine.
- *Bipolar electrode:* This 2-mm electrode uses bipolar energy and has to be used in combination with either nonionic media such as glycine or ionic media such as saline.
- *Bipolar Versapoint electrodes (Fig. 9):* These 2-mm electrodes use bipolar energy and have to be used in combination with Versapoint bipolar generator. These are of three types:
  1. Twizzle electrode

Hysteroscopic Morcellator (Fig. 11)

In 2005, the US Food and Drug Administration (FDA) approved the TruClear morcellator (Smith & Nephew, Andover, MA) as the first mechanical morcellator for intrauterine pathology.

In 2009, the FDA approved a second hysteroscopic morcellation device the MyoSure Tissue Removal System (Hologic, Bedford, MA). Like the first TruClear, the second-generation MyoSure system relies on a suction-based, mechanical energy, rotating tubular cutter system to remove intrauterine tissue. However, the newer MyoSure system has a smaller 2.5-mm inner blade that rotates and reciprocates within 3-mm outer tube at a speed as high as 6,000 rpm and presents an outer bevel rather than an inner bevel on the rotating blade edge. The blade and handpiece

Instruments for Hysteroscopy

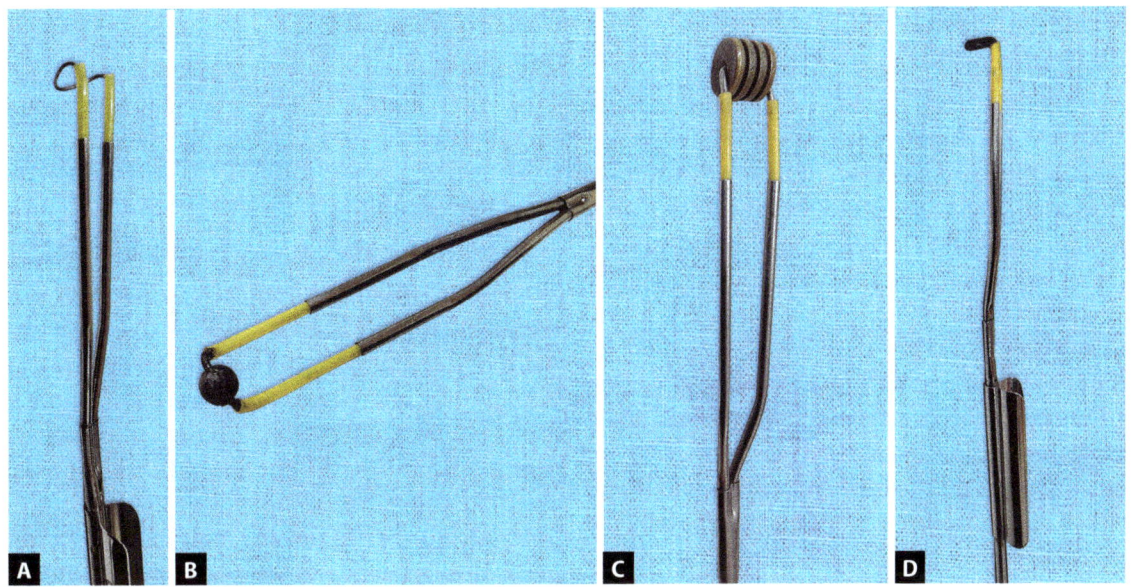

Figs. 10A to D: (A) Loop electrode; (B) Rollerball electrode; (C) Cylindrical electrode/Vaportrode; (D) Collins knife.

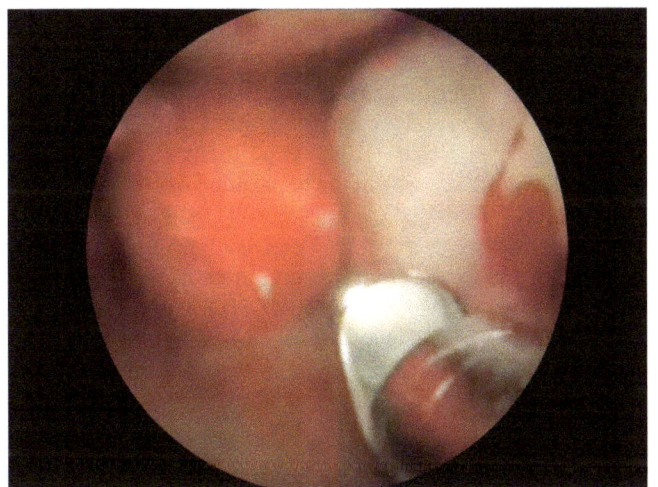

Fig. 11: Hysteroscopic morcellator.

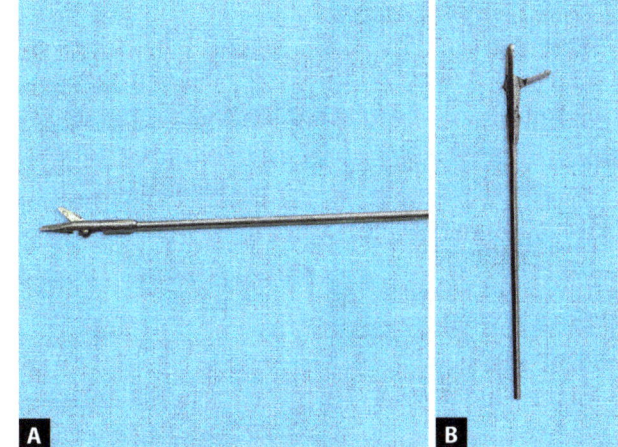

Figs. 12A and B: (A) Hysteroscopic scissors; (B) Hysteroscopic graspers.

are combined into a single-use device that is then attached to suction and a motor control unit. The device is introduced into the uterus through a 6.25-mm offset lens; custom-designed continuous flow hysteroscope that is compatible with all currently available fluid management systems.

Newer devices for hysteroscopic mechanical morcellation such as the Bigatti shaver (Karl Storz, GmBH, Germany) are being introduced into the market. Their performance vis-à-vis the first generation devices are yet to be evaluated.

Ancillary Instruments

These instruments can be rigid, semirigid, or flexible. The semirigid and flexible allow back and forth movement.

These instruments can be:
- Hysteroscopic scissors to cut adhesions or septum **(Fig. 12A)**
- Hysteroscopic grasping forceps **(Fig. 12B)**
- Hysteroscopic biopsy forceps
- Monopolar electrodes
- Bipolar electrodes

MAINTENANCE AND STERILIZATION OF INSTRUMENTS

After each operation, the reusable surgical instruments must be cleaned and sterilized. Collecting, decontaminating, and washing of the material are fundamental auxiliary procedures since the presence of organic residue seriously interferes with the sterilization process.

To that end, cleaning must only be undertaken after the instruments have been fully disassembled and immersed in warm water. One particularly useful tool for the preliminary phases is the water gun that generates a higher pressure than the faucet guaranteeing more thorough cleaning.

Utmost care must be taken when cleaning the lenses and scopes as these can be easily damaged. They should be washed with warm water; it is sometimes possible to use alcohol or special agents.

Endoscopes must be dried with cotton pledgets to avoid scratching the lenses. Upon completing these steps, any residual blurring can be removed using cotton balls soaked in 90% alcohol.

The fiberoptic light cable should be cleaned with special disinfectants and soapy water before being thoroughly rinsed. It is also important to inspect the light cable to make sure that the optical fibers are intact.

Biopsy forceps and scissors must also be subjected to cleaning, rinsing, drying, and lubrication.

Autoclave Sterilization

It is the cheapest system, and owing to the diffusion of steam, it cleans even the smallest gaps and openings. Only the optical systems and instruments which are specifically certified for the autoclave may be sterilized with a 20-minute cycle at 121°C or 7 minutes at 134°C.

Autoclave sterilization of endoscopes is a 20-minute cycle at 121°C or 7 minutes at 134°C. Autoclave sterilization of endoscopes requires certain special steps—they must be placed in a perforated metal container, wrapped in suitable gauze. It is better to allow natural cooling in order to prevent damage to the shafts. Certain steps are also necessary for the fiberoptic cables, such as arranging them in large loops to avoid twisting the bundles of fibers.

Gas Sterilization

Gas sterilization with ethylene oxide is an ideal system since it is performed at low temperatures obviating the risk of damaging the endoscopic instruments.

CONCLUSION

Hysteroscopy is to gynecology what cystoscopy is to urology. It is an absolutely invaluable part of the gynecologist's armamentarium. As one progresses in the field of gynecologic endoscopy, the gynecologist starts attempting and performing more and more complex procedures in hysteroscopy. However, before attempting these procedures, the gynecologist must be thoroughly aware of the instrumentation involved and its technical nuance. So that he or she can perform hysteroscopic procedures safely and with ease and master the art of troubleshooting in case of technical difficulties during use of these instruments.

REFERENCES

1. Moore JF, Carugno J. (2022). Hysteroscopy. [online] Available from: https://www.ncbi.nlm.nih.gov/books/NBK564345/. [Last accessed November, 2023].
2. Yen CF, Chou HH, Wu HM, Lee CL, Chang TC. Effectiveness and appropriateness in the application of office hysteroscopy. J Formos Med Assoc. 2019;118(11):1480-7.
3. Abdallah KS, Gadalla MA, Breijer M, Mol BWJ. Uterine distension media for outpatient hysteroscopy. Cochrane Database Syst Rev. 2021;11(11):CD006604.
4. Abdollahi Fard S, Mostafa Gharabaghi P, Montazeri F, Mashrabi O. Hysteroscopy as a minimally invasive surgery, a good substitute for invasive gynecological procedures. Iran J Reprod Med. 2012;10(4):377-82.
5. American College of Obstetrician and Gynecologist. (2020). The Use of Hysteroscopy for the Diagnosis and Treatment of Intrauterine Pathology. [online] Available from: https://www.acog.org/clinical/clinical-guidance/committee-opinion/articles/2020/03/the-use-of-hysteroscopy-for-the-diagnosis-and-treatment-of-intrauterine-pathology. [Last accessed November, 2023].
6. Kulkarni G, Shinde KK, Thosar M. Hysteroscopy: a boon in abnormal uterine bleeding. [online] Available from: https://www.ijrcog.org/index.php/ijrcog/article/view/6578. [Last accessed November, 2023].

3
Distension Media, Pressure System, and Electrosurgical Unit in Hysteroscopy

Shashikant Raghuwanshi, Rajesh Gajbhiye, Sandeep Nikhade

■ INTRODUCTION

Intrauterine surgery needs proper visualization. Distension of uterus and continuous irrigation is important for panoramic view of uterine cavity. For that, appropriate distension media and pressure systems play a key role. Electrosurgical unit is the core part of the operative hysteroscopy.

■ DISTENSION MEDIA

Normally the uterine cavity is collapsed, therefore appropriate distension is a must for proper visualization and to perform surgery. In order to achieve this, gaseous (carbon dioxide) and various liquid mediums are tried for distension of uterine cavity.

Ideal distension media has clear visibility, is isotonic, nonhemolytic, nonallergic, and provides ease at instrument use, cleaning, and with minimum impact on body fluids. It is easy to deliver, nonhemolytic, and nonconductive. Such medium in fact does not exist.

Fluid medium is preferably used over gaseous medium during hysteroscopy, as it gives clearer vision due to continuous irrigation and clear transparency.

Understandings of fluid dynamics are important as excessive fluid intravasation during hysteroscopy can lead to significant complications.

Types of distending fluids used are—either electrolyte containing (NS and RL) or nonelectrolyte containing (glycine and sorbitol) and its choice depends upon the type of energy is being used. For mechanical and bipolar current, NS and RL are used while for monopolar current, hypotonic glycine fluid is used. Monopolar current in electrolyte-containing solutions will lead to dispersion of current in media, reducing current density at focal area and hence heat generated will be insufficient to cause tissue effects.

Tissue removal systems refer to operative hysteroscopy that has been designed to simultaneously cut and aspirate tissue from within the uterine cavity. These systems usually incorporate their own fluid monitoring equipment but fluid overload can still occur.

■ TYPES OF DISTENSION MEDIA

Gaseous Distension Media

Carbon Dioxide

Carbon dioxide is the only gas recommended for uterine distension. It is commonly used in diagnostic hysteroscopy in the office setting. Carbon dioxide is not recommended for operative hysteroscopic procedures as the possibility of gas embolism is greatly increased as raw or ablated tissue provides the direct gas access to the uterine vasculature. CO_2 also mixes with blood to form froth that obscures' visibility of the operative field.

Fluid Distension Media

The advantage of fluid over gas is its ability to symmetrically distend the uterus with fluid and the ability to effectively flush blood, mucous, bubbles, and small tissue fragments out of the visual field giving more clearer visibility of operative field.

Types of liquid distension media are:
- *High-viscosity fluid:* Dextran 70 (Hyskon)
- *Low-viscosity fluids:*

Electrolytes (isotonic)	Nonelectrolytes
Normal saline	Glycine 1.5%
Ringer lactate	Sorbitol 3%
	Mannitol 5%
	Cytal—2.8% sorbitol + 0.5% mannitol

High-viscosity Fluid—Dextran 70 (Hyskon)

It is nonelectrolytic, nonconductive, minimally leaks through cervix and tubes providing excellent visibility. It is immiscible with blood. It being hyperosmolar largely expands plasma volume, causing massive fluid overload. It can produce anaphylactic reactions, pulmonary edema, acute respiratory distress syndrome (ARDS), coagulopathies, oliguria, and acute renal failure.

Isotonic Electrolyte-containing Solutions

The electrolyte-containing fluids are used in diagnostic and operative cases with mechanical, laser, or bipolar energy. Electrolytic solutions commonly used are normal saline and ringer lactate. These solutions are crystalloids which help to maintain the osmotic gradient between extravascular and intravascular compartments. While hyponatremia rarely occurs with normal saline or lactated ringer's solution, they more frequently cause isotonic fluid overload when intravasation occurs.

Characteristics of distension media used with procedures during hysteroscopy are given in **Table 1**.

Factors Affecting Fluid Absorption

Absorption of fluid into systemic circulation occurs through retrograde passage through fallopian tube, opening of vascular channels, and through endometrium. Factors that increase absorption are:
- Higher intrauterine pressure
- Longer duration of surgery—longer the procedure more is the time for fluid to get absorbed through various channels
- Deeper myometrial penetration
- Larger endometrial surface area
- General anesthesia is associated with rapid absorption of fluids and subsequent hyponatremia compared to local anesthesia. There might be delay in symptoms recognition in sedated patients.

Fluid Overload

There is no standard definition of fluid overload as data varies as per patient's age, medical fitness, and fluid deficit calculating systems. Incidence of fluid overload is around 5% in hysteroscopic procedure. Serum sodium drops by 10 mmol/L after absorption of 1,000 mL hypotonic 1.5% glycine. And that is the reason fluid absorption of 1,000 mL of hypotonic solution taken into consideration to define fluid deficit in a medically fit women of reproductive age group. For procedures using isotonic solutions fluid deficit of 2,500 mL is defined as fluid overload as per guidelines. Although upper limit depends upon patient's age and medical fitness. However, for patients with comorbidity such as cardiovascular diseases, renal impairment, lower threshold such as 750 mL for hypotonic and 1,500 mL for isotonic solutions should be used.

Factors impacting serious complications from fluid overload:
- *Osmolality of distension fluid:* Hypotonic electrolyte-free solutions such as glycine, mannitol, and sorbitol can cause hyponatremic hypervolemia. If unrecognized and left untreated, bradycardia and hypertension can develop, rapidly followed by pulmonary edema, cardiovascular collapse, and death.
- *Menopausal status:* Hyponatremia during hysteroscopy is especially problematic for premenopausal women, as they are at 25 time's greater risk for hyponatremic encephalopathy (HE) and permanent brain damage than postmenopausal women. Postmenopausal women developing dilutional hyponatremia are less likely to suffer brain damage because of their low estrogen and progesterone levels which allows there sodium pump to operate freely, as opposed to premenopausal patients, whose sodium pump is inhibited by higher levels of estrogen and progesterone.
- *Cardiovascular and renal disease:* These women are less likely to adapt sudden significant increases in intravascular fluid and land up in complication with lower fluid deficits.
- *How to reduce fluid absorption*

TABLE 1: Characteristics of distension media used with procedures during hysteroscopy.

Distension media	Electrolyte containing	Osmolality plasma—285 mOsm/L	Energy
Normal saline	Yes	285	Mechanical bipolar
Ringer's lactate	Yes	279	Laser
Glycine 1.5%	No	200	Monopolar
Dextrose 5%	No	Hypo-osmolar	Monopolar
Sorbitol 3%	No	165	Monopolar
Mannitol 5%	No	274	Monopolar
Dextran 32%	No		

- *Preoperative gonadotropin releasing hormone (GnRH) analog*
- *Intracervical vasopressin*
- *Low intrauterine pressure*—should be as low as possible for adequate visualization and below mean arterial pressure.
- *Use of suction devices*

Dilution Hyponatremia

More with hypotonic and electrolyte-free distension. Normal serum sodium is 135–142 mEq/L. Serum sodium <135 mEq/L can result in hyponatremia, which is categorized as mild, moderate, or severe. The first signs of hyponatremia can present with fluid deficits of 500 mL of hypotonic solution. Symptoms usually develop when serum sodium concentration drops below 125 mmol/L. In severe cases, permanent brain damage, coma, or death may result.

Slow intravenous (IV) infusion of 3% sodium chloride is given @ 1 mEq/L/h till it reaches to 125 mEq/L. This slow correction corrects cerebral edema and prevents osmotic demyelinating syndrome (central pontine myelinolysis). Hyponatremia below 120 mm/L should be treated with a 100 mL bolus of 3% saline over 10 minutes and this can be repeated up to three times, followed by an infusion as described above. The recommended target increase of the serum sodium is 6 mmol/L over 24 h until 130 mmol/L is reached.

Glycine Toxicity

Glycine by oxidative deamination splits into ammonia and glyoxylic acid. 2.2% glycine is isotonic 290 mosmol/L, risk of hyperammonemia is greater, and 1.5% of hypotonic glycine (200 mosmol/L) is clinically used. Fluid overload by glycine is hypervolemic hypo-osmolar hyponatremia.

Sorbitol Toxicity

Being hypo-osmolar (180 mosmol/L), it causes hypervolemic hyponatremia, hyperglycemia, and hypocalcemia. Myoclonus is presenting symptom. Treatment is with insulin on sliding scale with blood sugar monitoring and correction of hypocalcemia with 3 g calcium gluconate over 10 mins.

Fluid Overload with Isotonic Fluid Media

This medium reduces the risk of hypo-osmolarity and hyponatremia with excessive fluid absorption but does not eliminate the risk of congestive cardiac failure and pulmonary edema. Fluid restriction, diuretics, and monitoring are required.

■ DISTENSION SYSTEMS IN HYSTEROSCOPY

Intrauterine distension pressure can be maintained using simple gravity, manual, and automated pressure delivery systems.
- *Gravity systems* deliver the distension fluid by hydrostatic pressure. Elevation of the bag will increase the intrauterine pressure and one foot of height will give intrauterine pressure to around 25 mm Hg. When the fluid is maintained at a level of 5 feet above the patient's uterus, the intrauterine pressure will be between 70 and 100 mm Hg **(Fig. 1)**.
- *Manual pressure* systems maintain the necessary intrauterine pressure by using a pressure bag or blood pressure cuff around the fluid bag **(Fig. 2)**.

  The disadvantage of all these systems is that they keep the flow and the pressure at the inflow port constant and therefore if the pressure exceeds the mean arterial pressure, it can lead to excessive fluid absorption. Irrigation of fluid is achieved by opening partially or fully the outflow tap and applying varying amounts of negative pressure like suction from outflow tap.
- *Automated fluid pumps* will keep a constant pre-set pressure at the inflow port, but they will continue

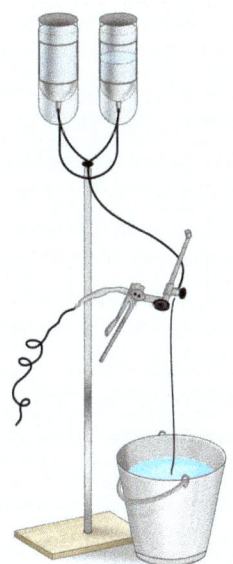

Fig. 1: Gravitation system.

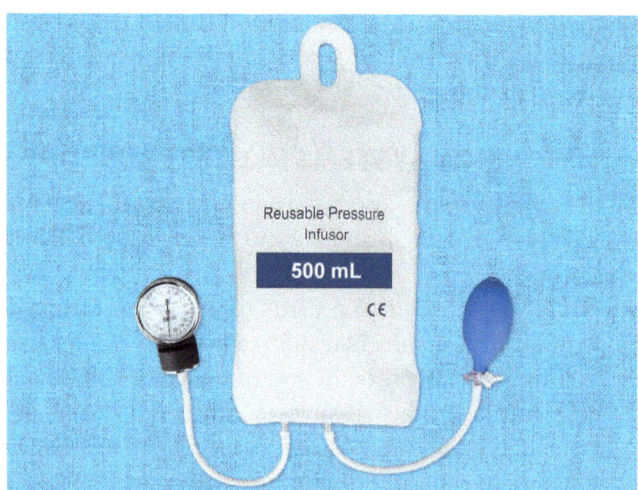

Fig. 2: Manual pressure system.

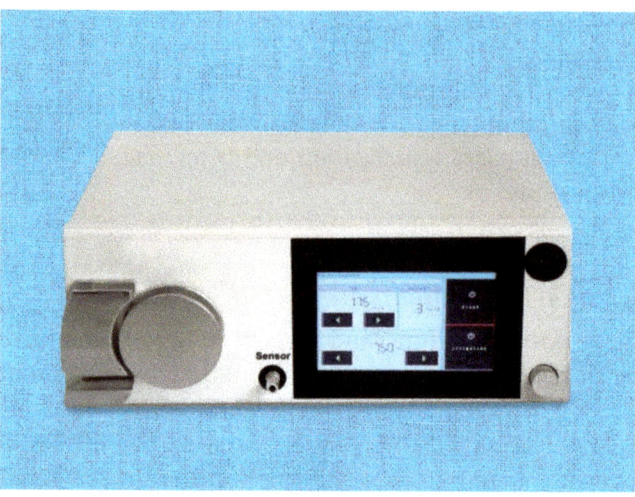

Fig. 3: Automated fluid pump.

delivering fluid despite the resistance in the uterine cavity. Other systems will titrate the intrauterine fluid pressure constantly at 70–80 mm Hg and will reduce the fluid flow (inflow and outflow) accordingly. Ideal device which maintains constant intrauterine pressure is more sensitive and limits excessive intrauterine pressures and subsequent intravasation of the distending medium. They are not necessary for short operative or diagnostic procedures but may be beneficial for prolonged, operative cases such as resection of the endometrium or submucosal fibroids where endometrial and myometrial disruptions occur causing bleeding and the formation of intrauterine tissue debris that can compromise visualization of the operative field **(Fig. 3)**.

- *The CO_2 tubal insufflator* delivers CO_2 at 30 mL per minute at pressure not exceeding 150 mm of Hg. The vacuum cannula is not used. Any leakage of gas is controlled by applying a Vulsellum laterally **(Fig. 4)**.

It is important that measurement and maintenance of the intrauterine pressure can be difficult when there is leakage of fluid around the cervix when cervical priming agents were used and when suction is applied at the outflow port of the hysteroscope.

Air or gas embolism is rare but can occur during a hysteroscopy with both gas (CO_2) or fluid distension media and in the outpatient as well as inpatient setting. Air can enter the uterine cavity during insertion of the hysteroscope if the inflow tubing is not primed with fluid or due to air bubbles within the distension medium potentially causing air embolism.

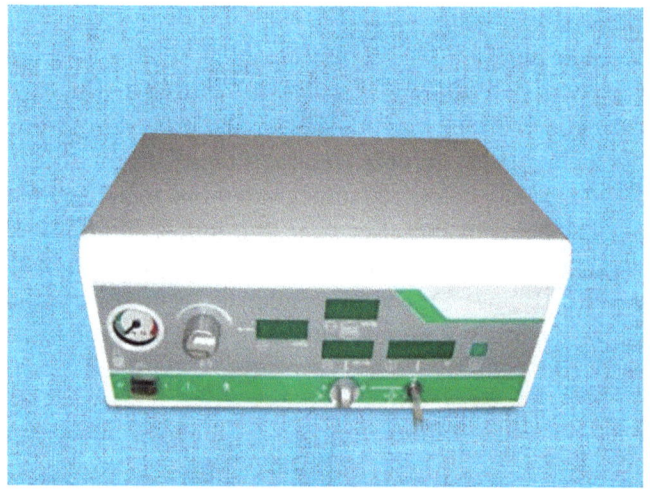

Fig. 4: CO_2 tubal insufflator.

To minimize the risk of air embolism, the hysteroscope and inflow tubing should be primed with the fluid media to eliminate air bubbles before inserting the hysteroscope into the uterine cavity.

ELECTROSURGICAL UNITS IN OPERATIVE HYSTEROSCOPY

To carry out operative hysteroscopy, we need to cut the tissue and control the bleeding. For this, we require energy in the form of electric current. Traditionally monopolar current was used for this **(Fig. 5)**. Here, the entire patient is involved in circuit and current passes through many tissues outside surgeons control, due to which there are greater chances of current diversion to undesirable locations.

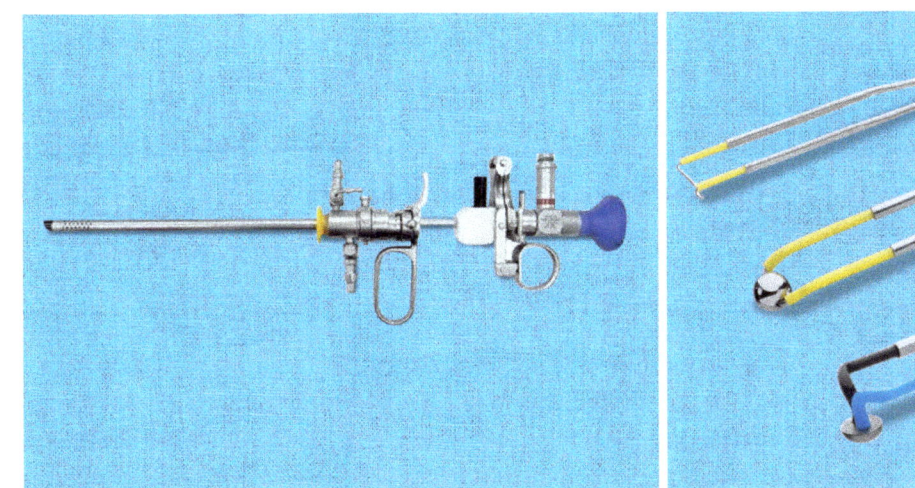

Fig. 5: Monopolar resectoscope with various electrodes.

In bipolar circuit on the other hand, current flows between two electrodes and the circuit is closed by placing tissue between two electrode and there is less chance of diversion. The risk of thermal injuries at distant organs or tissues, by direct contact of instruments, imperfection of insulation or diffusion of the electric current, is reduced in the bipolar technique.

The introduction of bipolar energy in the field of hysteroscopic surgery has meant the beginning of a new age of technology in which the best levels of security and effectiveness will be guaranteed. The main concerns in gynecological conventional monopolar resection are fluid absorption with hyponatremia, hypervolemia, and glycine toxicity. This syndrome is very dangerous for the patient, leading to neurotoxic coma and death in the worst cases. The bipolar hysteroscopic system has eliminated the need to use hypotonic solutions as irrigation medium, with its life-threatening complications. When limiting normal saline solution to 2 L, no serious complications associated with irrigation medium are expected. Most of the morbidities of the overflow syndrome are related to the use of hypotonic nonelectrolyte irrigation fluid. Furthermore, the risk of TUR syndrome is theoretically eliminated by using physiological sodium chloride solution for irrigation.

The bipolar resectoscope presents some advantages in comparison with the monopolar such as—better cut and coagulation by plasma effect of bipolar current, minor risks with the use of saline solution, lower alterations of the tissue, less bleeding during resection, better visibility, and reduced cost. The bipolar system is technically superior, cost-effective, and safer in comparison with the monopolar system.

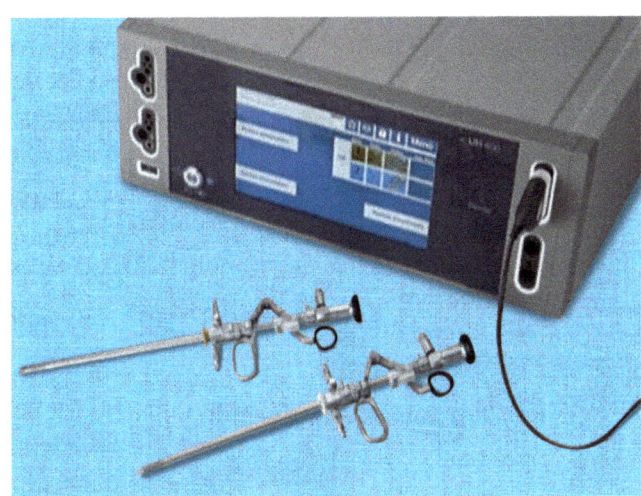

Fig. 6: *Bipolar resectoscope:* It has a cutting loop similar to traditional resectoscopes.

As active and the return electrodes are placed on the resectoscope, high current densities are achieved locally and complications caused by distant negative effects of the current are theoretically reduced in vivo. High-frequency current generated by a bipolar instrument tends to remain superficial furthermore, the coagulation capacity by itself is extremely more powerful in the bipolar system in comparison with monopolar. This avoids time-consuming recoagulation after resection for coagulation and contributes to close the superficial capillary vascularization, also reducing intravasation.

In bipolar electrodes, active and the return electrodes are placed on the resectoscope **(Figs. 6 and 7)**.

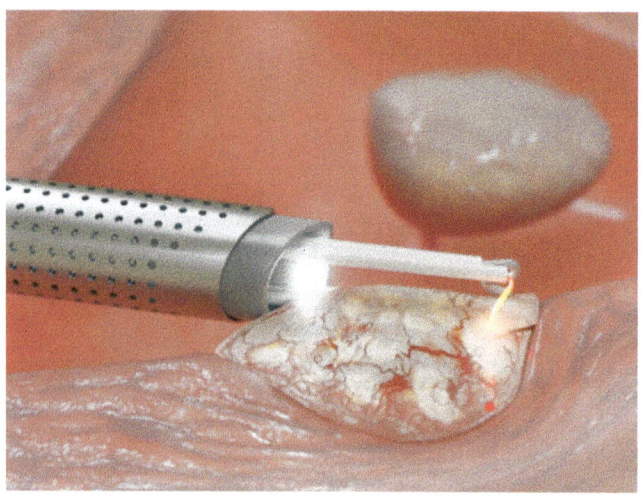

Fig. 7: Bipolar resectoscopy for myoma. Type II leiomyoma: Dense tissue, vasculature at base.

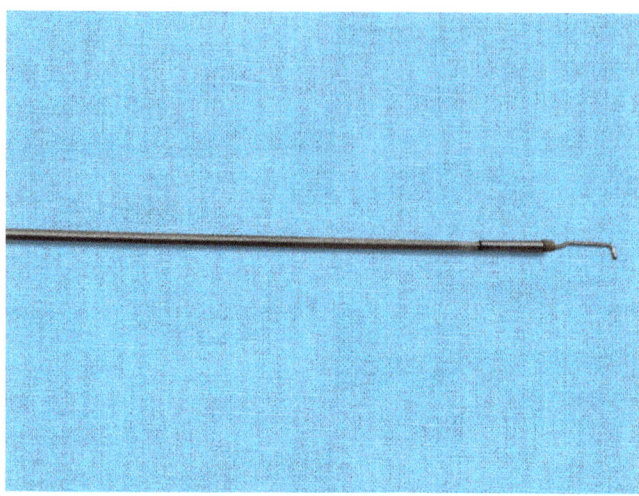

Fig. 8: Bipolar hook electrode.

Types of bipolar electrodes are spring, twizzle, and ball electrode.
- Spring tip is used for hemostatic vaporization of large areas.
- Ball tip for precise vaporization
- Twizzle tip for hemostatic resection and morcellation of tissue.

Hook electrode and needle type bipolar electrodes are very cost-effective and good for septum resection and intrauterine adhesiolysis **(Fig. 8)**.

Uses:
- Removal of submucous fibroids
- Transection of intrauterine septa
- Removal of polyps
- Endometrial ablation
- Transection of intrauterine adhesions.

CONCLUSION

Thus, bipolar electrodes and resectoscopes have the advantages of using saline as a distension media which prevents major risk associated with glycine toxicity. The bipolar system is technically superior and cost-effective.

Office Hysteroscopy

Chapter 4

Nitin Shah, Aditi Joshi Godbole

INTRODUCTION

Hysteroscopy is considered as the gold standard for diagnosis as well as treatment of intrauterine pathologies and at times for cervical pathologies as well. With the advent in technology, smaller diameter telescopes are now available. In addition, the availability of distension media in the form of normal saline has made office hysteroscopy an attractive and safe option for patient care, decreasing the burden of hospital admissions.

Common indications for office hysteroscopy include:
- Targeted endometrial sampling in cases of abnormal uterine bleeding (AUB)
- Removal of impacted intrauterine contraceptive device
- Retained products of conception
- Small polyps
- Pre-IVF (in vitro fertilization) evaluation and treatment
- Myomectomy (selected cases)
- Second look hysteroscopy.

PREPARATION OF PATIENT

Office hysteroscopy provides the advantage of doing the procedure on an OPD basis, eliminating the anxiety and fear associated with the operation room for the patients. Counseling forms the crux of patient preparation. A proper detailed explanation of the procedure must be done prior to the procedure. It is extremely important to solve all the queries and alleviate any fears that the patient may have regarding the procedure.

Ideally, the appropriate time to post for the surgery is within a week of cessation of menses (Days 5–11) to enable good visualization and avoid the problems of navigation and visibility due to endometrial growth in the latter part of the cycle.[1]

Salient features in preoperative preparations:
- Proper valid written informed consent
- Give a dose of injectable anticholinergic like atropine (0.6 mg intramuscular) or glycopyrrolate (0.2 mg intramuscular) half hour prior to procedure to avoid sudden vasovagal attacks.
- Analgesia is not mandatory. However in case of nulliparous, perimenopausal women or in anxious patients, an oral painkiller may be given 1–2 hours prior to the procedure.
- Cervical preparation is usually not required, unless the patient is premenopausal or has a stenotic cervix. In these cases, instillation of vaginal prostaglandin E1 analog like misoprostol 200–400 mg 12 hours prior to the procedure can minimize the pain associated with cervical manipulation in these patients.

It is extremely important to keep conversing with the patient while performing the procedure to keep them engaged and distracted.[2]

PREPARATION OF SURGEON

The operating surgeon must keep the operating trolley well equipped and set prior to start the procedure. There are various types of telescopes available, rigid as well as flexible ones. The rigid telescopes are usually preferred. The basic set up comprises a small rigid diagnostic telescope with an outer sheath (approximate diameter of 2.9–4 mm). The telescope has a fore-oblique view which helps to negotiate the internal os readily since it is oval in shape. The sheath has an inflow and outflow channel which in turn is connected to an irrigation system. It also has an operative channel that will allow for passing certain instruments for small procedures.

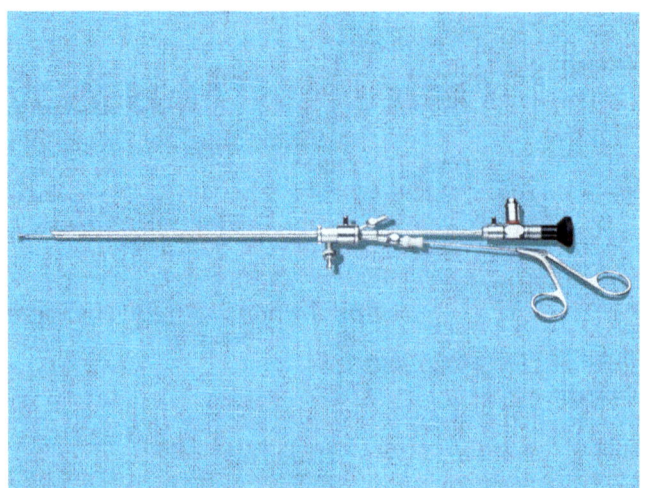

Fig. 1: Rigid hysteroscope with outer sheath and operating channel.

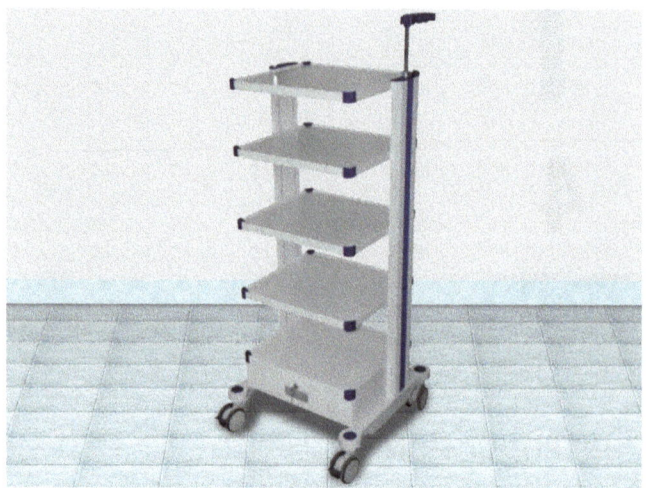

Fig. 3: Equipment cart.

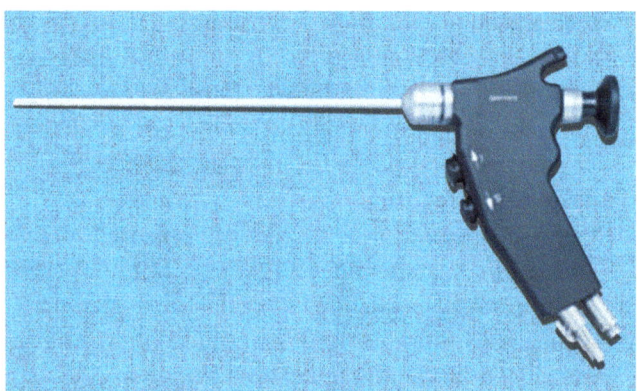

Fig. 2: BETTOCCHI Integrated Office Hysteroscope telescope.

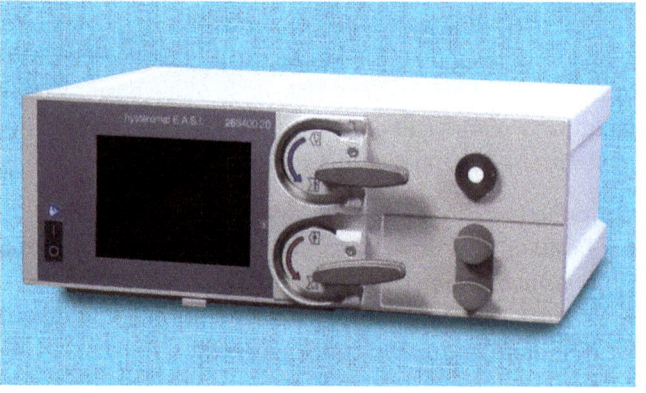

Fig. 4: Hysteromat.

There is also a BIOH (BETTOCCHI Integrated Office Hysteroscope) telescope, which has a continuous flow system, with a total diameter of 4 mm **(Figs. 1 and 2)**. It has two sheaths, one for irrigation and one for suction. Few other types of scopes which are available for office hysteroscopy include TROPHYscope or CAMPO compact hysteroscope and versa scope.

Furthermore, there is an equipment cart which has a monitor, light source, camera, and camera-connecting unit **(Fig. 3)**. There are especially designed irrigation units available called hysteromat which regulate intrauterine pressure more accurately, however for office procedures even a manual air pump with handcuff can be used around the distension media bottle to provide the necessary pressure but must be used with caution **(Fig. 4)**.

Keep additional instruments on a secondary trolley if anticipating any therapeutic procedures like polypectomy or adhesiolysis. Make sure you have a prior pelvic ultrasound done before the procedure to avoid last minute surprises. In addition, you may keep a syringe filled with local anesthesia, vaginal speculum, anterior vaginal wall retractor, sponge-holding forceps, and some gauze pieces. The patient is placed on the examination table in lithotomy position which enables easy manipulation.

During the procedure, keep two assistants, one to regulate the pressure of the inflation bag and other to help with the instruments at the trolley. Assemble your scope prior to start the procedure. Make sure there is a plastic collection bag near the foot end of your examination table to collect the outflow water coming from the vagina to prevent spillage on the floor.

Always enter via the vaginoscopic approach which avoids instrumentation and manipulation of the cervix. Once you enter the cervix and reach the internal os, wait patiently for the os to dilate by the pressure of the distension media to avoid pain associated with negotiation of internal os.[3]

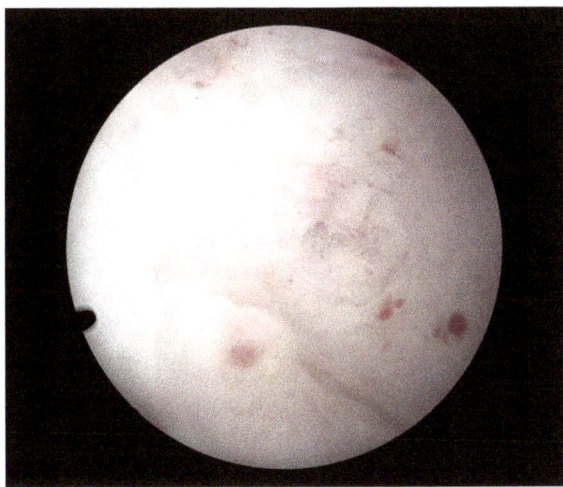

Fig. 5: Tuberculosis endometritis.

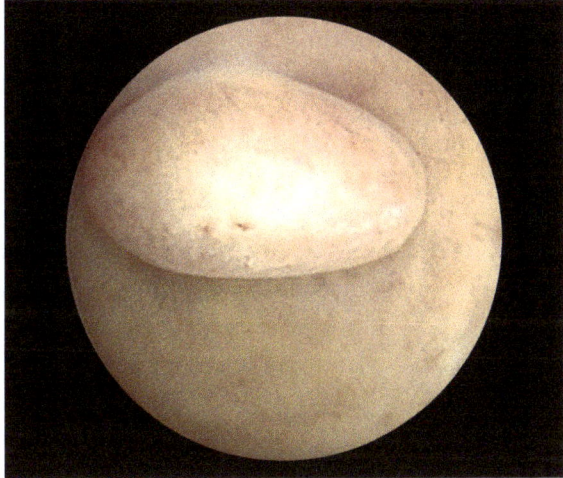

Fig. 6: Uterine polyp.

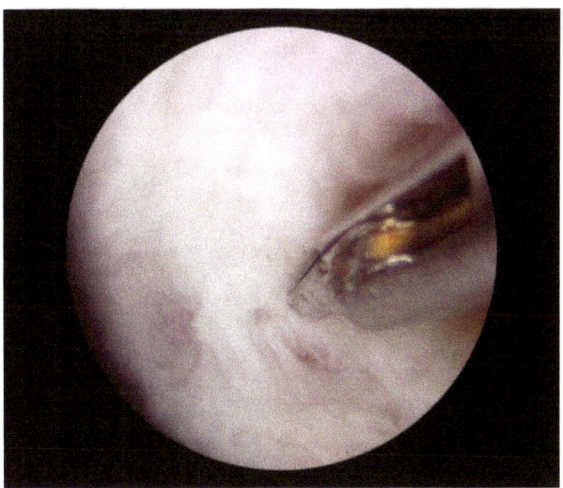

Fig. 7: Asherman's syndrome.

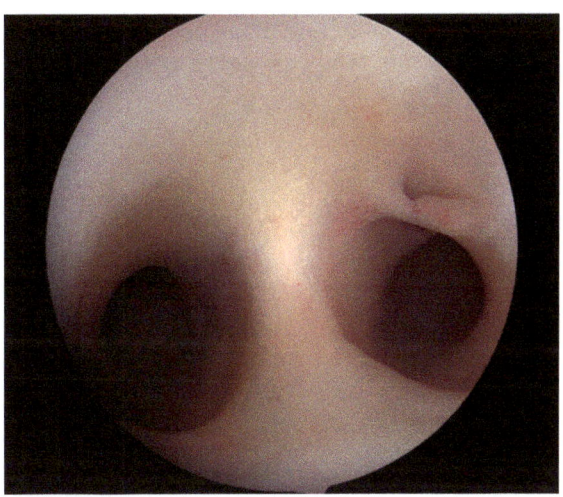

Fig. 8: Septal resection.

Which instrument and when

Operating scissors: These are small 3 or 5 Fr instruments that can be introduced from the working channel of the scope. They are preferred for taking biopsy in tubercular endometritis, cutting small septum, adhesions, and polypectomy. Centralize the lesion and the proceed with the dissection **(Figs. 5 to 8)**.

In expert hands, a myoma <1 cm can also be tackled during an office hysteroscopy. The base of the myoma is cut with a scissor, and the myoma is held with a tenaculum and entire assembly is removed together.

Operating graspers: These are 3/5 Fr instruments which have a blunt end. They enable us to grasp small polyps and avulse them from the base. They can also be utilized for obtaining an endometrial sample for targeted biopsies which is way superior to a blind dilatation and curettage in cases of abnormal uterine bleeding. They are also useful for retrieving a misplaced intrauterine device and at times even for removal of retained products of conception **(Figs. 9 and 10)**.

Advancement in newer resectoscope equipments has enabled the use of electrosurgery in case of thick septum, dense adhesions, or small myomas. A mini Gubbini resectoscope (16 Fr) of 5 mm diameter is now available that bypasses the need for cervical dilatation which is needed with the traditional 26-Fr Gubbini resectoscope **(Fig. 11)**.[4]

The introduction of newer hysteroscopic tissue removal systems such as Truclear, Myosure, and IBS with a modern fluid management system is also an emerging

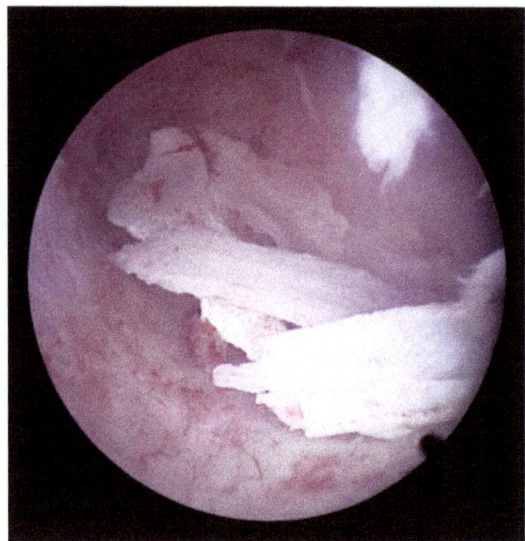

Fig. 9: Osseous metaplasia.

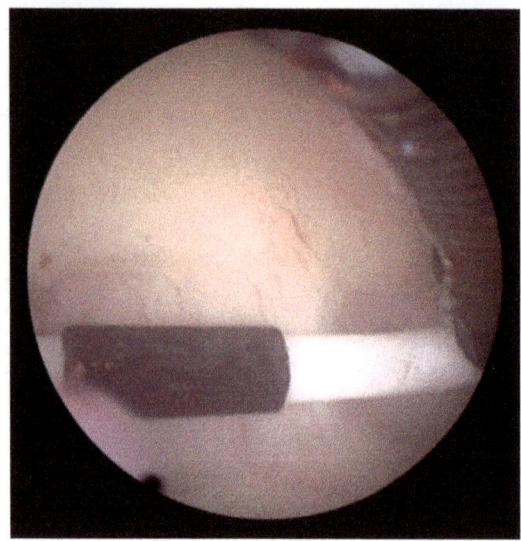

Fig. 10: Retained intrauterine device.

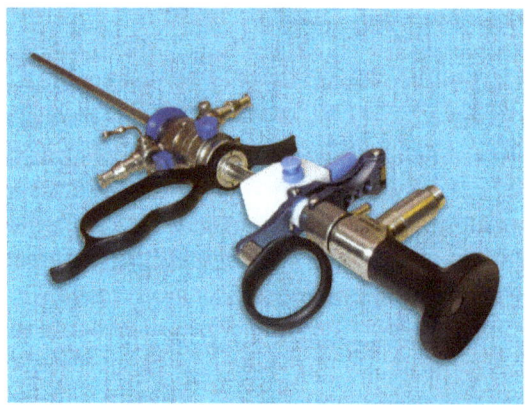

Fig. 11: Mini Gubbini resectoscope.

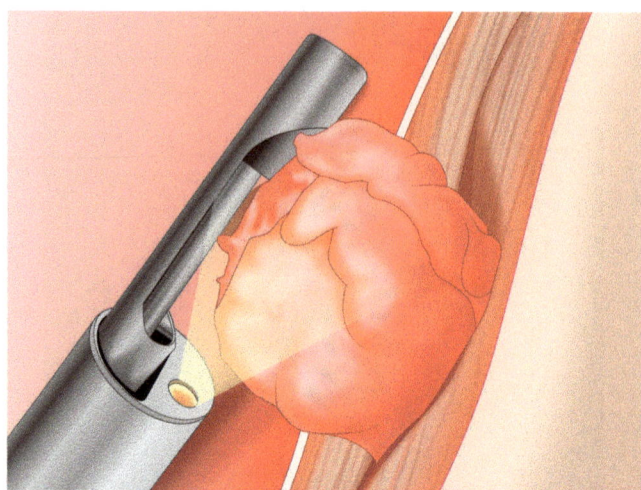

Fig. 12: Hysteroscopic tissue removal system.

option for office-based management of intrauterine pathologies. However, these systems are expensive and have a certain degree of learning curve associated with it. More randomized trials are needed to compare its equivalence and effectiveness with the mini resectoscopes **(Fig. 12)**.

SMART TIPS FOR OFFICE HYSTEROSCOPY

- Always keep your trolley ready with the instruments required.
- Keep a nursing staff near the patient's head to communicate and observe the patient.
- Preferably do diagnostic procedures immediately after cessation of menses to enable good visualization.
- Prefer the vaginoscopic approach for hysteroscopy. This eliminates need to hold the cervix.
- Keep pressure of distension media around 45 mm Hg to avoid discomfort to the patient due to uterine distension.
- Do not touch the myometrium while performing the scopy to avoid pain for the patient.
- Operating scissors must have a sharp cutting edge to enable easy and quick dissection of the tissue.

CONCLUSION

Office hysteroscopy is the gold standard for visualization of uterine pathologies and offers the "see and treat" option. It enables us to have an accurate diagnosis as well provides an opportunity to treat the pathologies at the same setting. It is a cost-effective, easy, and a safe procedure, although it does have a certain degree of a learning curve.

TAKEAWAYS

- Office hysteroscopy is gaining popularity; however, it requires a certain degree of skill and training.
- Analgesia in form of local anesthesia can be given especially whenever performing any operative hysteroscopy procedures.
- Vaginoscopic approach eliminates the need to hold the cervix. Thus making the procedure more patient's friendly.
- A mini Gubbini resectoscope has now made it feasible to do selected therapeutic cases on OPD basis, which need electrosurgical equipment.
- It is a cost-effective and safe procedure.

REFERENCES

1. Salazar CA, Isaacson KB. Office Operative Hysteroscopy: An Update. J Minim Invasive Gynecol. 2018;25(2):199-208.
2. Pados G, Makedos A. Office Hysteroscopy [Internet]. Endoscopy - Innovative Uses and Emerging Technologies. InTech; 2015.
3. Mairos J, Di Martino P. Office Hysteroscopy. An operative gold standard technique and an important contribution to Patient Safety. Gynecol Surg. 2016;13:111-4.
4. Haimovich S, Kumar A, Salazar S, Hanstede M. (2022). The Mini-Recsectoscope: A Real Innovation or Just Another Trend? [online] Available from: https://newsscope.aagl.org/volume-36-issue-8/spotlight-on-hysteroscopy/. [Last accessed November, 2023].

Chapter 5

Endometrial Polyp: How to Deal with it?

Sergio Haimovich, Tanvir Singh

INTRODUCTION

Endometrial polyps (EPs) are structural abnormalities of the uterus.[1] They are single or multiple well-circumscribed, localized lesions of different size and shape protruding in the endometrial cavity. Their size varies from millimeters to centimeters. They contain endometrium stroma, glands, fibrous tissue, and blood vessels.[2] The overall prevalence of EPs is 8–35%.[3,4] EPs are usually asymptomatic, but when symptomatic, they present as abnormal uterine bleeding and can contribute to infertility.[5] The prevalence of cancer in EP is 2.7%.[6] This chapter aims at describing the ethology and different types of polyps, and operative tips for their management.

ETIOLOGY[7]

- Obesity (unopposed estrogen)
- Diabetes mellitus
- Hypertension
- *Women on tamoxifen:* Risk of recurrence in high
- Advancing age
- There is a possibility of endometrial cancer driver mutations in EPs, when there is no menstrual shedding.[8]

Histological types of EP are:[9]
- Functional
- Atrophic
- Hyperplastic
- Myomatous
- Mixed
- Adenomatous
- Malignant transformation

DIAGNOSIS

Endometrial polyps are diagnosed by following modalities:[10]

- *Pelvic ultrasonography:* 2D and 3D with power Doppler
- Sonohysterography
- Hysterosalpingography
- *Hysteroscopy:* Gold standard for diagnosis and treatment of polyps

TREATMENT (TABLE 1)

Asymptomatic polyps: Endometrial polyps are usually asymptomatic and benign, and expectant management is acceptable in these situation, when the polyps are small (maximum diameter <10 mm) and single. They regress in 30% of cases.[11]

Symptomatic polyps: Hysteroscopy is the gold standard for the evaluation and treatment of EPs.

Hysteroscopic polypectomy can be performed with or without anesthesia in the office, outpatient, or operating theater.[10]

Hysteroscopic tissue removal system (HTRS) was found to have the shortest operative time and fastest learning curve.[15]

When treating for abnormal uterine bleeding, recurrence rate is found to be lower when polypectomy is combined with endometrial resection.[16]

Risk of recurrence is high when the largest diameter of polyp is >10 mm.[11]

Polypectomy is associated with lowest risk of complications (0.95%).

DISCUSSION AND CONCLUSION

No one instrument is superior over the other. The choice of instrument depends on multiple factors:
- Infrastructure
- Availability of the equipment
- Expertise of the surgeon

Endometrial Polyp: How to Deal with it?

TABLE 1: Comparing different techniques.

Instrument	Scissors + grasper (Figs. 1A to D)	Grasper (Figs. 2A to C)	Electrode needle (Figs. 3A to C)	Laser (Figs. 4A to D)	Hysteroscopy tissue removal system (Figs. 5A to C)	Mini resectoscope (Figs. 6A and B)	Resectoscope (Figs. 7A to C)
Size of instrument	5 Fr with 4 and 5 mm hysteroscopy	5 Fr with 4 and 5 mm hysteroscopy	5 Fr with 4 and 5 mm hysteroscopy	5 Fr with 4 and 5 mm hysteroscopy	5 mm/6 mm and 8 mm	15 Fr/16 Fr	22/26 Fr
Energy source	Mechanical	Mechanical	Bipolar	Diode/CO_2/Nd:YAG	Mechanical	Bipolar/monopolar/plasma	Bipolar/monopolar/plasma
Technique	Cut the base with scissors + retrieve with grasper	Grasping the base of the polyp and pushing it forward	Slicing the polyp and retrieve with grasper	Slicing the polyp and retrieve with grasper	Cutting and suction action	Slicing technique and remove with the loop electrode	Slicing technique and remove with the loop electrode
Setting	Office/outpatient/operating theater	Office/outpatient/operating theater	Office/outpatient/operating theater	Office/outpatient/operating theater	Office/outpatient/operating theater	Office/outpatient/operating theater	Operating theater
Reusability	Reusable	Reusable	Reusable	Disposable	Reusable/disposable	Reusable/disposable	Reusable/disposable
Fluid media	Normal saline	Normal saline	Normal saline	Normal saline	Normal saline	Normal saline/glycine	Normal saline/glycine
Polyp number	Easier in single	Easier in single	Easier in single	Easier in single	Single/multiple	Single/multiple	Single/multiple
Polyp size	No restriction	No restriction	No restriction	No restriction	No restriction	No restriction	No restriction
Polyp recurrence	5%[12]	15%[12]		2.2%[13]		0–13%[14]	0–13%[14]

(Nd:YAG: neodymium-doped yttrium aluminum garnet)

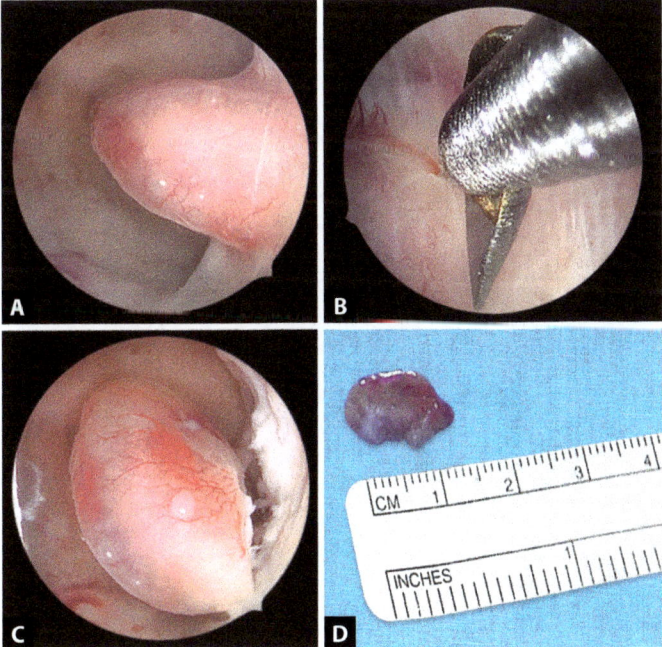

Figs. 1A to D: *Single sessile polyp:* (A) Attached to the left lateral wall; (B) 5 Fr scissors is used to excise the polyp from the base, inserted through a 5-mm hysteroscopy using a 12° scope; (C and D) The excised polyp is removed with 5 Fr alligator forceps.

Courtesy: Images by Dr Tanvir Singh.

26 Endometrial Polyp: How to Deal with it?

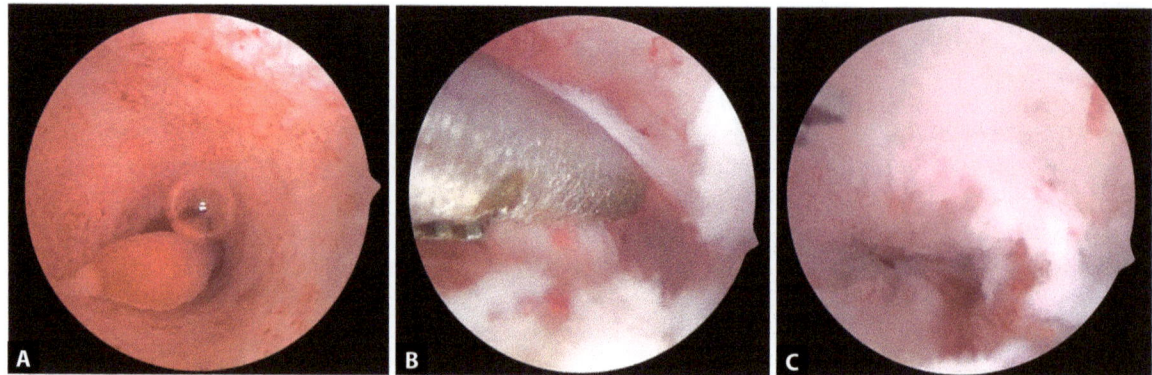

Figs. 2A to C: (A) Ostia polyp; (B) Excised with 5 Fr alligator forceps; (C) Postexcision, postal opening seen.
Courtesy: Images by Dr Tanvir Singh.

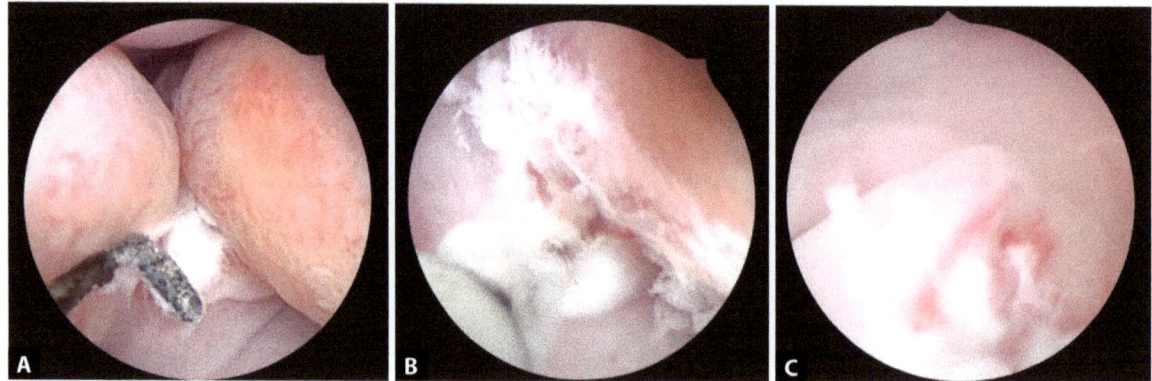

Figs. 3A to C: Vaginal polyp treated with (A), (B) 5 Fr electrode bipolar needle; (C) Base of the polyp.
Courtesy: Images by Dr Tanvir Singh.

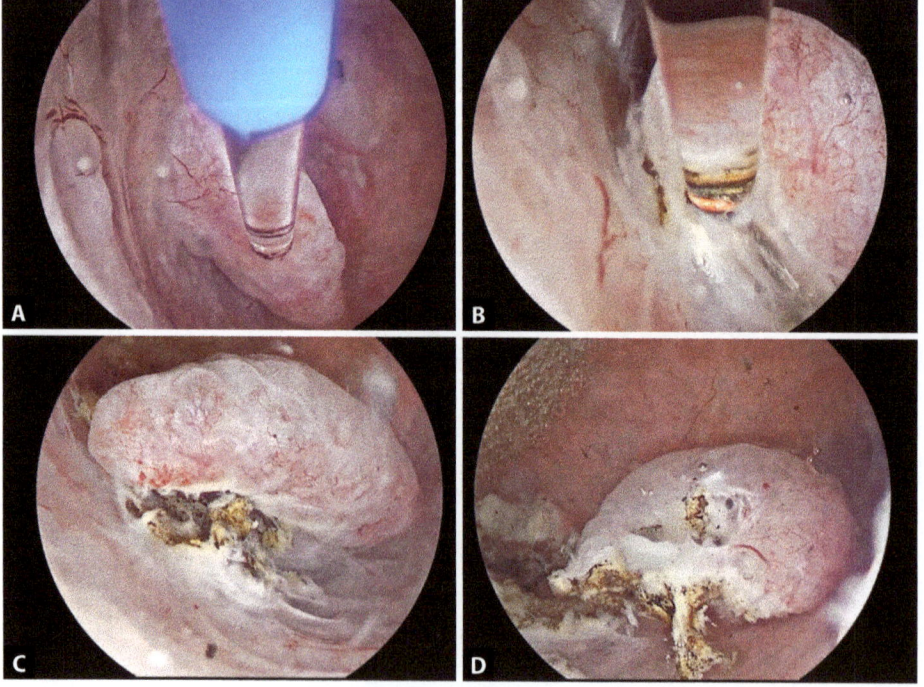

Figs. 4A to D: Polyp removed with diode laser.

Endometrial Polyp: How to Deal with it?

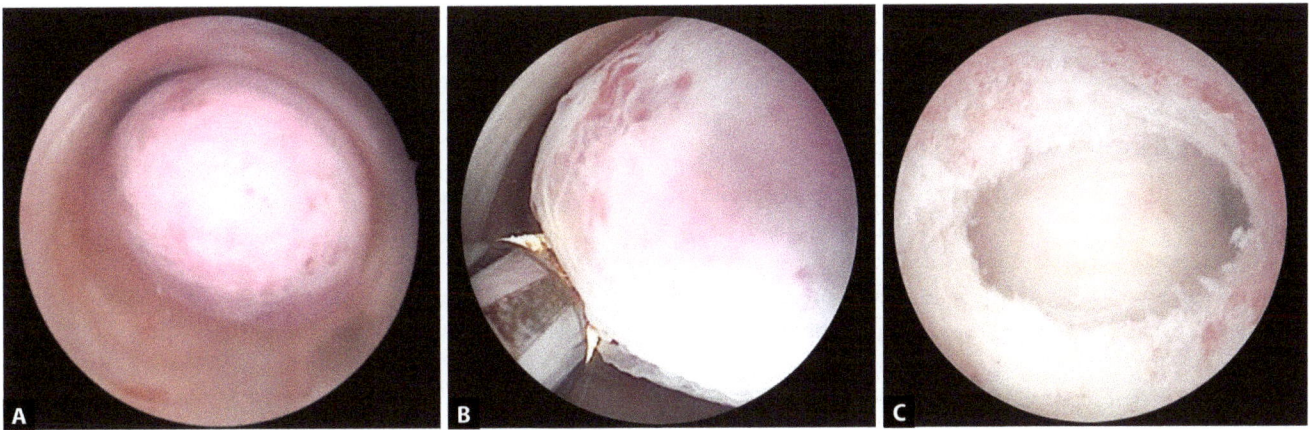

Figs. 5A to C: (A) Polyp removed using hysteroscopic tissue removal system; (B) TruClear Elite 6 mm is with incisor insert is used. It has a 5 mm window with oscillatory action to cut and aspirate the tissue at the same time; (C) Visual dilatation and curettage performed the endometrium following polyp removal.
Courtesy: Images by Dr Tanvir Singh.

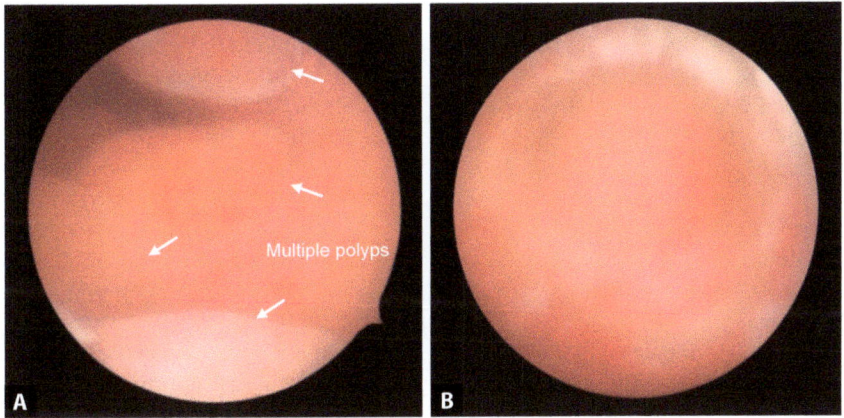

Figs. 6A and B: (A) Multiple polyps removed with TruClear Elite in office; (B) Hysteroscopic polypectomy followed by visual dilatation and curettage performed.
Courtesy: Images by Dr Tanvir Singh.

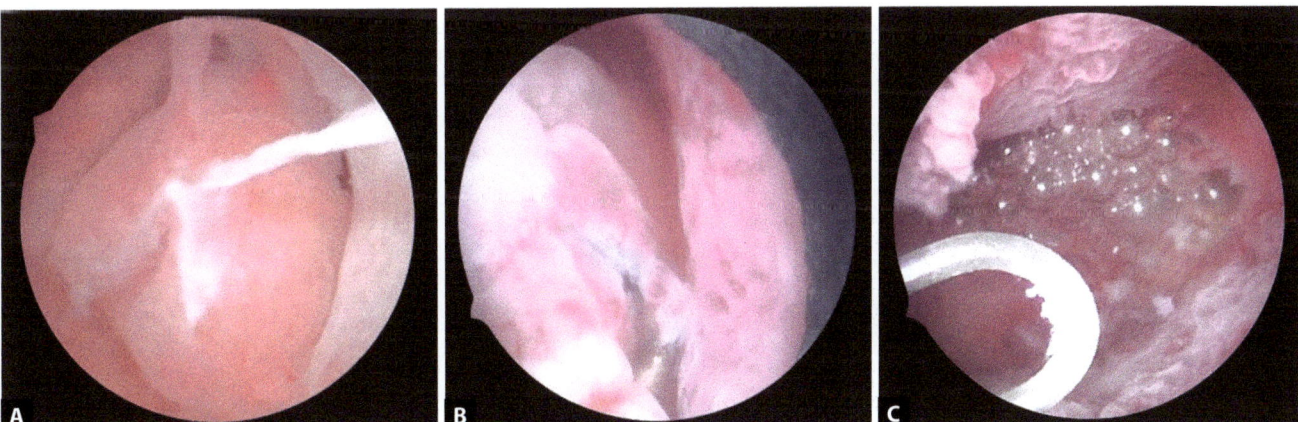

Figs. 7A to C: (A) Polyp close to left ostia; (B) 16 Fr Gubbini resectoscope with bipolar loop electrode is seen in the picture; (C) Slicing technique is used to excise the polyp.
Courtesy: Images by Dr Tanvir Singh.

- Cost-effectiveness
- Indication of surgery—either infertility or abnormal uterine bleeding

Combining ultrasonography with power Doppler studies prior to hysteroscopy gives an added advantage to understand the location, number, size, and the vascularity of the polyps, including the risk of probable malignancy. Depending on the risk factor profile of the patient, polyps removal must be followed by the biopsy of the underlying endometrium.[8] Office hysteroscopic polypectomy offers advantage of low cost to the patient, high patient satisfaction, feasible, no hospital admission, and reduces overall healthcare costs.

REFERENCES

1. Munro MG. Uterine polyps, adenomyosis, leiomyomas, and endometrial receptivity. Fertil Steril. 2019;111(4):629-40.
2. Ludwin A, Lindheim SR, Booth R, Ludwin I. Removal of uterine polyps: clinical management and surgical approach. Climacteric. 2020;23:388-96.
3. Valentin L. Re: Prevalence of endometrial polyps and abnormal uterine bleeding in a Danish population aged 20-74 years. Ultrasound Obstet Gynecol. 2009;33:369-70; author reply 370.
4. American Association of Gynecologic, L. AAGL practice report: practice guidelines for the diagnosis and management of endometrial polyps. J Minim Invasive Gynecol. 2012;19:3-10.
5. Perez-Medina T, Bajo-Arenas J, Salazar F, Redondo T, Sanfrutos L, Alvarez P, et al. Endometrial polyps and their implication in the pregnancy rates of patients undergoing intrauterine insemination: a prospective, randomized study. Hum Reprod. 2005;20:1632-5.
6. Uglietti A, Buggio L, Farella M, Chiaffarino F, Dridi D, Vercellini P, et al. The risk of malignancy in uterine polyps: a systematic review and meta-analysis. Eur J Obstet Gynecol Reprod Biol. 2019;237:48-56.
7. Serhat E, Cogendez E, Selcuk S, Asoglu MR, Arioglu PF, Eren S. Is there a relationship between endometrial polyps and obesity, diabetes mellitus, hypertension? Arch Gynecol Obstet. 2014;290(5):937-41.
8. Sahoo SS, Aguilar M, Xu Y, Lucas E, Miller V, Chen H, et al. Endometrial polyps are non-neoplastic but harbor epithelial mutations in endometrial cancer drivers at low allelic frequencies. Mod Pathol. 2022;35(11): 1702-12.
9. Malpica A, Deavers MT, Euscher ED. Biopsy interpretation of the uterine cervix and corpus. Philadelphia, USA: Biopsy Interpretation Series, Wolters Kluwer Health-Lippincott Williams & Wilkins; 2009. pp. 169-75.
10. Raz N, Feinmesser L, Moore O, Haimovich S. Endometrial polyps: diagnosis and treatment options—a review of literature. Minim Invasive Ther Allied Technol. 2021;30(5):278-87.
11. Bohîlțea RE. Diagnosticul patologiei endometriale. București, Romania: Universitară "Carol Davila"; 2018. pp. 71-177.
12. Preutthipan S, Herabutya Y. Hysteroscopic polypectomy in 240 premenopausal and postmenopausal women. Fertil Steril. 2005;83:705-9.
13. Perino A, Castelli A, Cucinella G, Biondo A, Pane A, Venezia R. A randomized comparison of endometrial laser intrauterine thermotherapy and hysteroscopic endometrial resection. Fertil Steril. 2004;82:731-4.
14. Paradisi R, Rossi S, Scifo MC, Dall'O' F, Battaglia C, Venturoli S. Recurrence of endometrial polyps. Gynecol Obstet Invest. 2014;78:26-32.
15. Smith P, Middleton L, Connor M, Clark TJ. Hysteroscopic morcellation compared with electrical resection of endometrial polyps: a randomized controlled trial. Obstet Gynecol. 2014;123:745-51.
16. Vahdat M, Mousavi AS, Kaveh M, Sadegi K, Abdolahi H. Hysteroscopic polypectomy with endometrial resection preventing the recurrence of endometrial polyps: A single-blinded randomized clinical trial. Caspian J Intern Med. 2022;13(2):393-7.

Chapter 6

Septum and Management Plan

Tanvir Singh

■ INTRODUCTION

Uterine septum represents 35% of congenital uterine malformations (CUMs). It is the most common form.[1,2] Uterine septum has abnormal blood supply, increased muscle in the septum leading to uncoordinated uterine contractions, and decreased number of glandular and ciliated cells in the endometrium. These factors increase the risk of infertility, implantation failure, recurrent miscarriage, and obstetrical complications.[3,4]

■ CLASSIFICATION AND TYPES

Two main classification systems are: (1) American Society for Reproductive Medicine—ASRM [(American Fertility Society (AFS)] classification initially published in 1988, which was subsequently modified in 2016 and 2021, and (2) the European Society of Human Reproduction and Embryology (ESHRE)/European Society for Gynaecological Endoscopy (ESGE) Working Group classification devised in 2014. **Table 1** expands on the details and comparison of both classifications.

The CONgenital UTerine Anomalies (CONUTA) ESHRE/ESGE Working Group defined a septate uterus as a congenital uterine anomaly with pathological persistence of the median septum due to an abnormal resorption phenomenon, a normal outline of the uterine fundus.[5] This category is further divided into two subclasses (U2a and U2b), depending on whether the apex of the septum reaches the internal cervical os or stops above it[6] (**Fig. 1**).

■ PLANNING

In asymptomatic women, diagnosed septum must be documented (**Figs. 2A and B**). (European Society of Gynaecological Endoscopy). Should hysteroscopy metroplasty be performed?

This is one of the most controversial discussions. There are no randomized clinical trials to answer the question of whether metroplasty should be offered to patients with septum in primary infertility, especially prior to in vitro fertilization (**Figs. 3A to C**). The main indication for surgical removal of septum is poor obstetric outcome (**Figs. 4A to C**).

A systemic review and meta-analysis from 2022 found that uterine septum had a detrimental effect on pregnancy rate, live birth rate, spontaneous abortions, and pregnancy loss. After septum removal, the proportion of live birth rate was higher [odds ratio (OR) 49.58, 95% confidence interval (CI) 29.93-82.13; $p < 0.0001$] and the proportion of spontaneous abortion and pregnancy loss was lower after the removal of the septum (OR 0.02, 95% CI 0.02-0.04; $p < 0.000$ and OR 0.05, 95% CI 0.03-0.08; $p < 0.0001$)[3] (**Figs. 5 and 6**).

European Society of Human Reproduction and Embryology, National Institute of Health and Care Excellence (NICE), and the Royal College of Obstetricians and Gynaecologists (RCOG) are not in favor of treating a septum for infertility.

TRUST (The Randomised Uterine Septum Trial) concluded the septum resection does not improve reproductive outcomes. Though this is a multicenter study including 10 centers, the limitations were the low sample size of 80, and the study lasted for a decade, and subgroup analysis of live birth rate, preterm birth, spontaneous abortion, recurrent pregnancy loss, and infertility was not possible.[7,8]

■ OPERATIVE TIPS

Hysteroscopic metroplasty (HM) is preferably performed in the early proliferative phase. It can be performed in the

TABLE 1: Features of ASRM and ESHRE–ESGE classification.

ASRM[6]	ESHRE–ESGE
2021	Working group—CONUTA (CONgenital UTerine Anomalies) devised the guideline in 2016
Based on the American Fertility Society (AFS) classification. It is simple, reproducible	Based on the anatomy of female genital tract
It includes all categories of anomalies to improve clinical care	Anomalies are grouped based on clinical significance
Uses descriptive words, such as uterus didelphys, duplicated cervix, with obstructed right hemivagina and right renal agenesis	Uses terms such as U3 C2 V2 or VCUAM (V5a, C1, U2, A0, MR)
Describes the various anomalies and the variations of the uterus, cervix, and vagina. It has a more detailed diagrammatic representation of the variants of the anomalies	Describes the various anomalies and the variations of the uterus, cervix and vagina
Provides user with surgical or medical options	
Gynecological examination should be performed	Gynecological examination should be performed
Ideal screening tool: Ultrasound or magnetic resonance imaging (MRI)	*Diagnostic tool and accuracy in decreasing order:* 3D US (97.6%), sonohysterography (SHG; 96.5%), 2D US (86.6) and hysterosalpingography (HSG; 86.9%). MRI (90%)
Ideal diagnostic tool: MRI, during imaging, either by ultrasound or MRI, it is good to evaluate for aplastic or ectopic kidney	3D US may be more accurate than MRI in sub-classifying malformations
	Uterine wall thickness is the reference point to differentiate between dysmorphic T-shaped, septate and bicorporeal uteri
Ultrasound measurement in coronal plane with visible intramural parts of the tubal ostia. Septate uterus: Fundal indentation of <1 cm and internal fundal indentation of >1.5 cm	• Ultrasound measurement in sagittal plane at the thickest part. Uterine wall thickness is the reference point • *Septate:* Internal fundal indentations >50% of the uterine wall, and the depth of the external intercornual cleft was <50%
Possible risk of underdiagnosis	Possible risk of overdiagnosis of septate uterus

(ASRM: American Society for Reproductive Medicine; ESGE: European Society for Gynaecological Endoscopy; ESHRE: European Society of Human Reproduction and Embryology)
Source: Pfeifer SM, Attaran M, Goldstein J, Lindheim SR, Petrozza JC, Rackow BW, et al. (2021). ASRM mullerian anomalies classification 2021. [online] Available from: https://www.asrm.org/globalassets/_asrm/practice-guidance/practice-guidelines/pdf/mac2021_manuscript.pdf. [Last accessed November, 2023].

operating theater or in office setting. Progesterone therapy can be administered prior to surgical correction to thin the endometrium.

Hysteroscopically, uterus is inspected starting from a panoramic view and visualizing both the ostia. Keeping both the tubal ostia under vision as a guiding point, a transverse incision is given in the midline of the septum. This helps to avoid injury to the healthy myometrium. The fundal thickness is maintained at 10–15 mm.

The procedure is considered complete when both the ostia are visualized in a panoramic view with free side to side movement of the hysteroscope.

Uterine perforation usually occurs at the posterior wall, when the correct plane of incision is lost. Traditionally, prior to advent of miniaturized instruments, HM was performed with 26-Fr or 22-Fr resectoscope using Collin's knife. These required cervical dilatation with Hegar's dilators. Now, HM can be performed using 5-Fr instruments via 4- or 5-mm hysteroscope or 16-Fr mini-resectoscope in office or operating room.

CONCLUSION

Follow-up ultrasound with a relook hysteroscopy can be performed to know the success of the procedure. Patient must always be counseled for a two-step procedure. We do know that treating the septum improves reproductive and obstetric of both partial and complete septum. Though data is limited, HM should be offered to women with recurrent pregnancy loss and infertility.

Septum and Management Plan

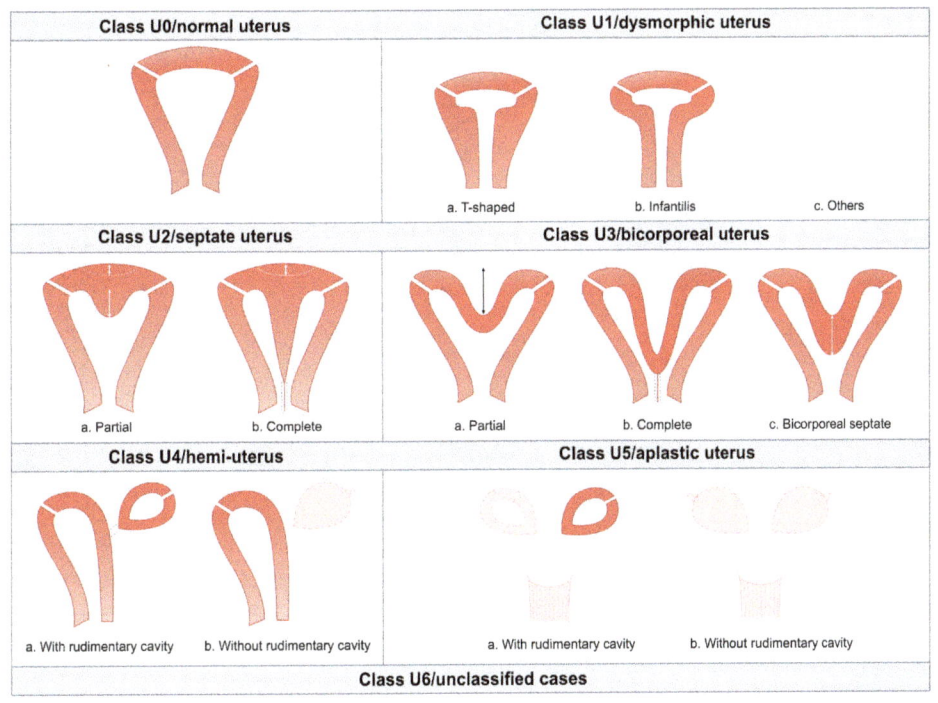

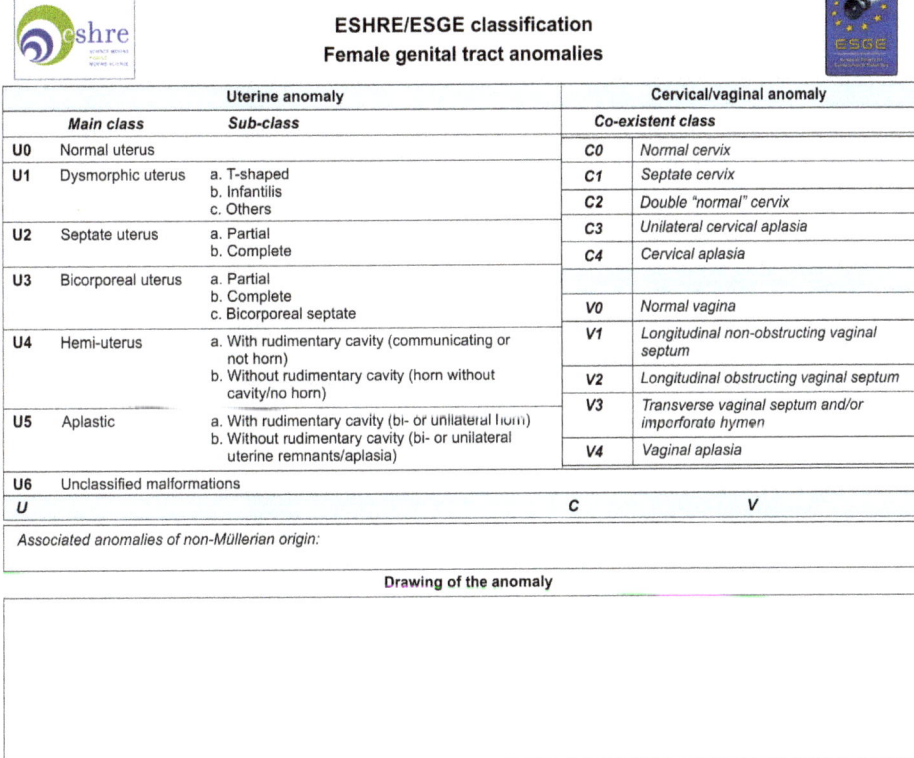

Fig. 1: *ESHRE/ESGE classification of uterine anomalies:* Schematic representation (Class U2: internal indentation, 50% of the uterine wall thickness and external contour straight or with indentation, 50%, Class U3: external indentation, 50% of the uterine wall thickness, Class U3b: width of the fundal indentation at the midline, 150% of the uterine wall thickness). (ESGE: European Society for Gynaecological Endoscopy; ESHRE: European Society of Human Reproduction and Embryology)

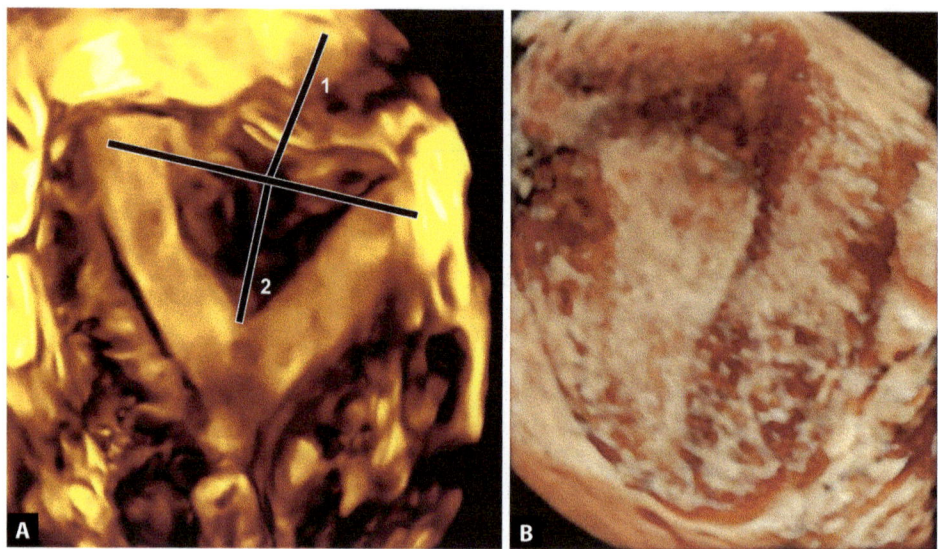

Figs. 2A and B: Complete septum. (A) 3D transvaginal ultrasound (TVS) view of a complete septate uterus: 1—uterine wall thickness: distance between the line joining tubal ostia (interostial line) and a parallel line on the top of uterine fundus, 2—internal midline indentation: distance between the interostial line and a parallel line on the top of midline indentation (the line reaches the internal cervical os); (B) Follow-up 3D TVS view following resection of complete septum.

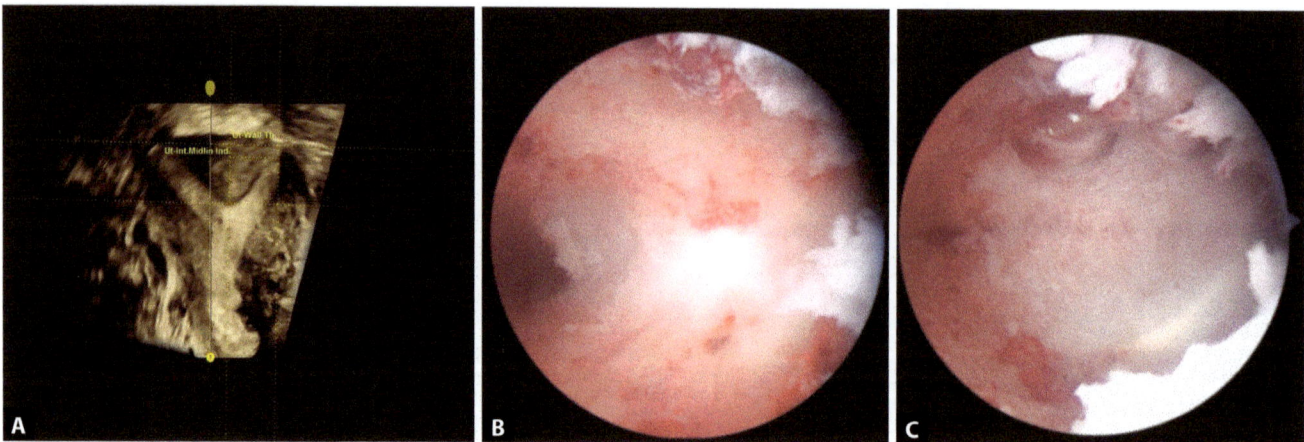

Figs. 3A to C: (A) Partial septum; (B) Hysteroscopic view of partial septum; (C) Hysteroscopic view of partial septum following of excision.

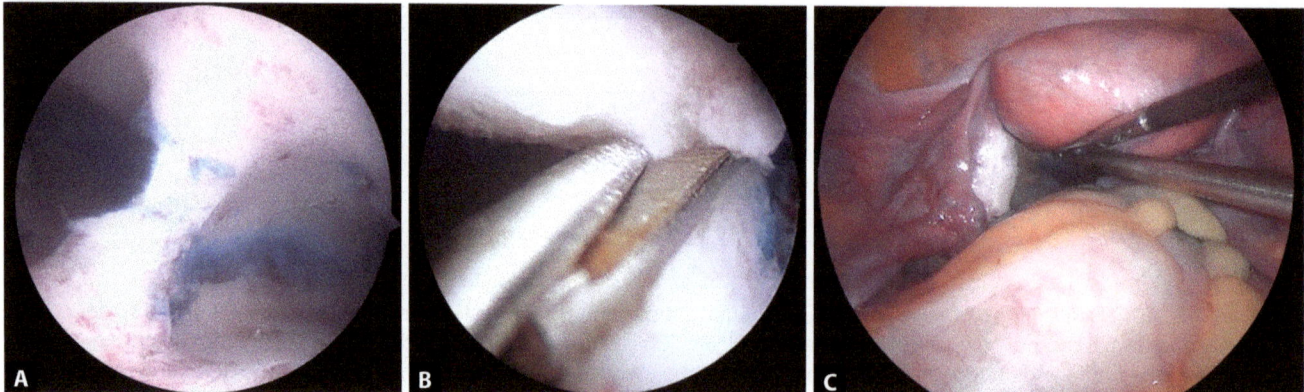

Figs. 4A to C: (A) Hysteroscopic view of partial septum following methylene blue test; (B) Partial septum, cut with scissors; (C) Laparoscopic view of flattened broad fundus in septum.

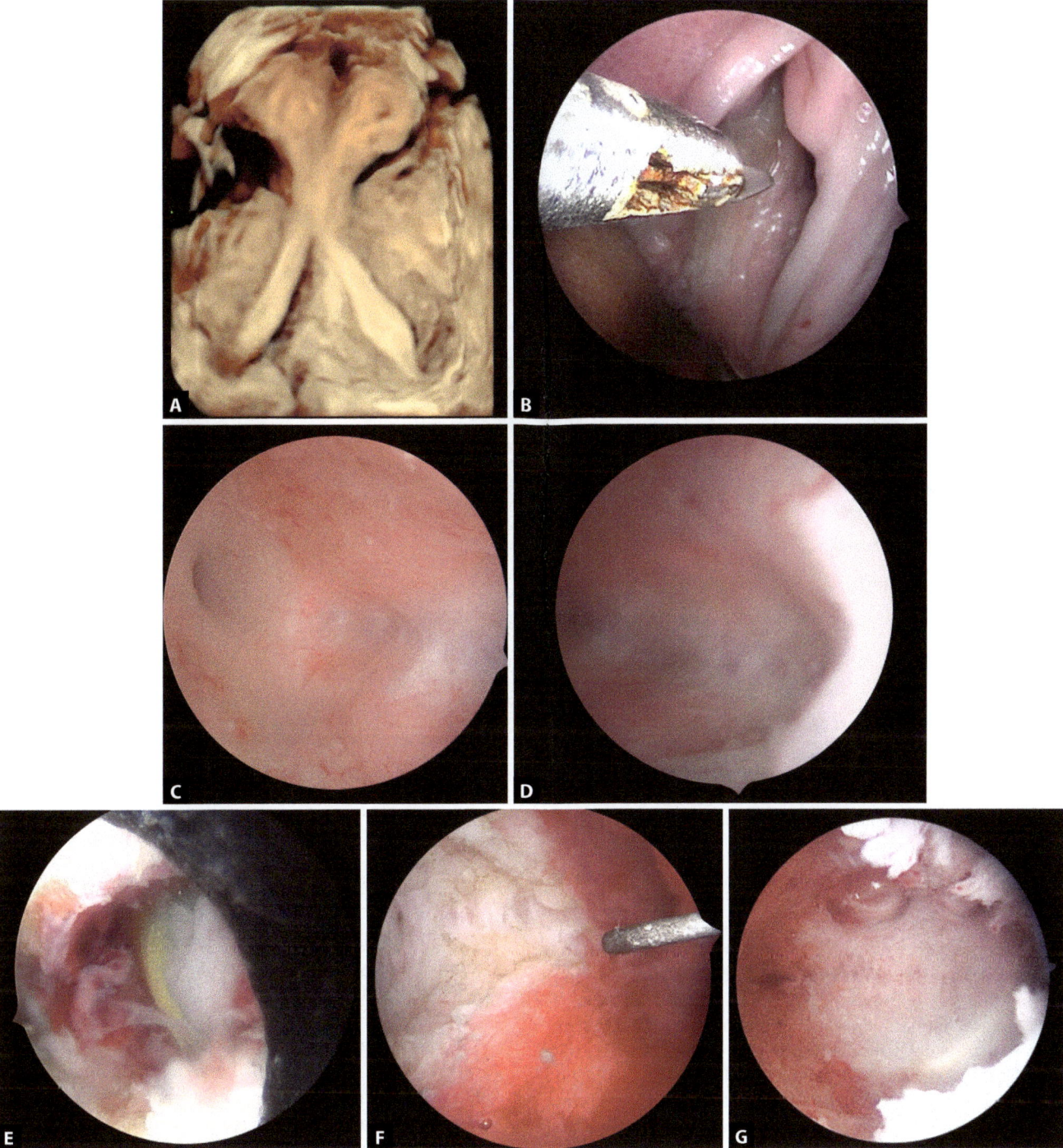

Figs. 5A to G: (A) Transvaginal ultrasound picture of complete septum with double cervix and vaginal septum; (B) Vertical vaginal septum, cut with 5-Fr hysteroscopic scissors; (C) Hysteroscopic view of left ostia; (D) Hysteroscopic view of right ostia; (E) 6-Fr Foley's catheter placed in the right side of the septum. An incision is made with a Collin's knife of 16-Fr mini-resectoscope from the left side just above the internal os in the midline until the catheter bulb is seen; (F and G) Hysteroscopic view following septal selection.

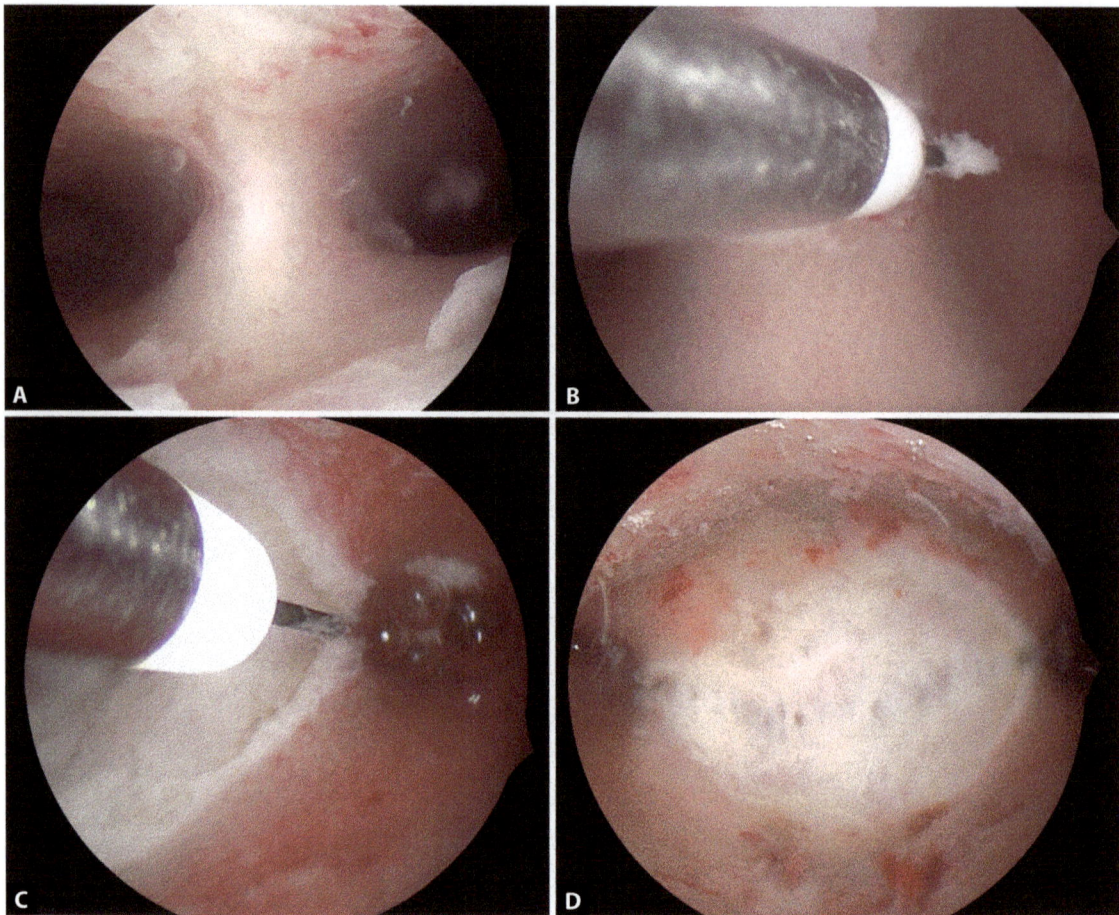

Figs. 6A to D: (A) Hysteroscopic view of partial septum; (B) Hysteroscopic excision of partial septum using bipolar electrode needle. Incision is taken in the midline keeping the ostia as the reference point; (C) Septum is excised until both ostia are visualized; (D) Final view after septum resection.

REFERENCES

1. Hollett-Caines J, Vilos GA, Abu-Rafea B, Ahmad R. Fertility and pregnancy outcomes following hysteroscopic septum division. J Obstet Gynaecol Can. 2006;28:156-9.
2. Grimbizis GF, Camus M, Tarlatzis BC, Bontis JN, Devroey P. Clinical implications of uterine malformations and hysteroscopic treatment results. Hum Reprod Update. 2001;7:161-74.
3. Noventa M, Spagnol G, Marchetti M, Saccardi C, Bonaldo G, Laganà AS, et al. Uterine septum with or without hysteroscopic metroplasty: impact on fertility and obstetrical outcomes—a systematic review and meta-analysis of observational research. J Clin Med. 2022;11:3290.
4. Chang Y, Shen M, Wang S, Guo Z, Duan H. Reproductive outcomes and risk factors of women with septate uterus after hysteroscopic metroplasty. Front Endocrinol. 2023;14:1063774.
5. Grimbizis GF, Di Spiezio Sardo A, Saravelos SH, Gordts S, Exacoustos C, Van Schoubroeck D, et al. The Thessaloniki ESHRE/ESGE consensus on diagnosis of female genital anomalies. Gynecol Surg. 2016;13:1-16.
6. Pfeifer SM, Attaran M, Goldstein J, Lindheim SR, Petrozza JC, Rackow BW, et al. ASRM müllerian anomalies classification 2021. Fertil Steril. 2021;116(5):1238-52.
7. Rikken JFW, Kowalik CR, Emanuel MH, Bongers MY, Spinder T, Jansen FW, et al. Septum resection versus expectant management in women with a septate uterus: an international multicentre open-label randomized controlled trial. Hum Reprod. 2021;36(5):1260-7.
8. Ludwin A, Ludwin I. Comparison of the ESHRE-ESGE and ASRM classifications of Müllerian duct anomalies in everyday practice. Hum Reprod. 2015;30(3):569-80.

Mullerian Anomalies Other than Septum: Role of Hysteroscopy

Chapter 7

Ashish Kale

INTRODUCTION

Rare developmental malformations of the female reproductive system are known as Mullerian anomalies. Nearly 5% of unselected people are thought to have Mullerian abnormalities, but uterine anomalies afflict women with reproductive problems more frequently, with prevalence rates of 8% in infertile women and 13% in women with a history of miscarriage, respectively.[1] There have been several efforts to categorize conditions affecting the paired Mullerian ducts and define certain categories of abnormalities based on morphologic similarity, embryologic origin, clinical consequences, and suitable therapy. Hysteroscopy can play a significant role in the diagnosis and management of nonseptate Müllerian duct anomalies (MDAs), which are congenital uterine abnormalities that result from incomplete development of the Mullerian ducts during fetal development.[2] These anomalies can affect a woman's reproductive health and may lead to various gynecological issues.

TYPES AND ETIOLOGY

The American Society for Reproductive Medicine (ASRM) Mullerian Anomalies Classification 2021 classifies Mullerian anomalies into nine categories: (1) Mullerian agenesis, (2) cervical agenesis, (3) unicornuate uterus, (4) uterus didelphys, (5) bicornuate uterus, (6) septate uterus, (7) longitudinal vaginal septum, (8) transverse vaginal septum, and (9) complex anomalies. Please refer to **Figure 1** for detailed insights. The exact etiology of MDAs is not fully understood, but they are believed to result from disruptions or abnormalities in the embryological development of the Müllerian ducts.[3] The Müllerian ducts are the precursors to the female reproductive organs, including the uterus, fallopian tubes, and upper part of the vagina. Here are some factors that may contribute to the etiology of MDAs:[4]

- *Genetic factors:* Genetic mutations or variations in specific genes involved in the development of the Müllerian ducts may play a role in the development of these anomalies. Research has identified potential candidate genes associated with MDAs.
- *Hormonal factors:* Hormonal imbalances during fetal development may interfere with the normal differentiation and fusion of the Müllerian ducts. Hormonal disturbances can disrupt the proper development of the female reproductive organs.
- *Environmental factors:* Exposures to certain environmental factors or teratogens during pregnancy may contribute to the development of MDAs. These factors can include exposure to toxins, drugs, or infections during critical periods of embryonic development.
- *Multifactorial causes:* MDAs are likely influenced by a combination of genetic, hormonal, and environmental factors. The interplay of these factors can lead to a wide range of anomalies with varying severity.
- *Unknown factors:* In some cases, the exact cause of Mullerian duct anomalies remains unknown. The complexity of embryological development and the potential for multiple contributing factors make it challenging to pinpoint a single cause.

DIAGNOSIS OF MULLERIAN ANOMALIES

Diagnostic techniques that can evaluate the entire pelvis, uterus, including the myometrium, internal uterine structure, and communications between specific parts of the female tract [ultrasound, magnetic resonance imaging (MRI)] can be divided from those that are primarily focused on the uterine cavity [hysteroscopy and hysterosalpingography (HSG)], pelvis, and external uterine structure (laparoscopy), or only the uterine cavity.[5]

In the past, laparoscopy and hysteroscopy were regarded as the gold standard for uterine anomaly diagnosis and categorization.[6]

■ SURGICAL APPROACH

For the correction of anomalies, there have been technological advances in surgical equipment's that led to development of minimal invasive techniques.[5] The intrauterine cavity and ostia can be directly seen during hysteroscopy. As a result, it is particularly effective in detecting congenital uterine defects and is frequently used to provide a firm diagnosis following an aberrant HSG results **(Fig. 2)**. However, it does not allow for the assessment of the uterus's exterior shape, making it frequently insufficient for discriminating between various abnormality kinds. As a result, more research is necessary to accurately distinguish between bicornuate and septate uteri, most frequently a diagnostic laparoscopy. Hysteroscopy with laparoscopy offers the added advantage of concurrent treatment, as in the case of a uterine septum resection.[7]

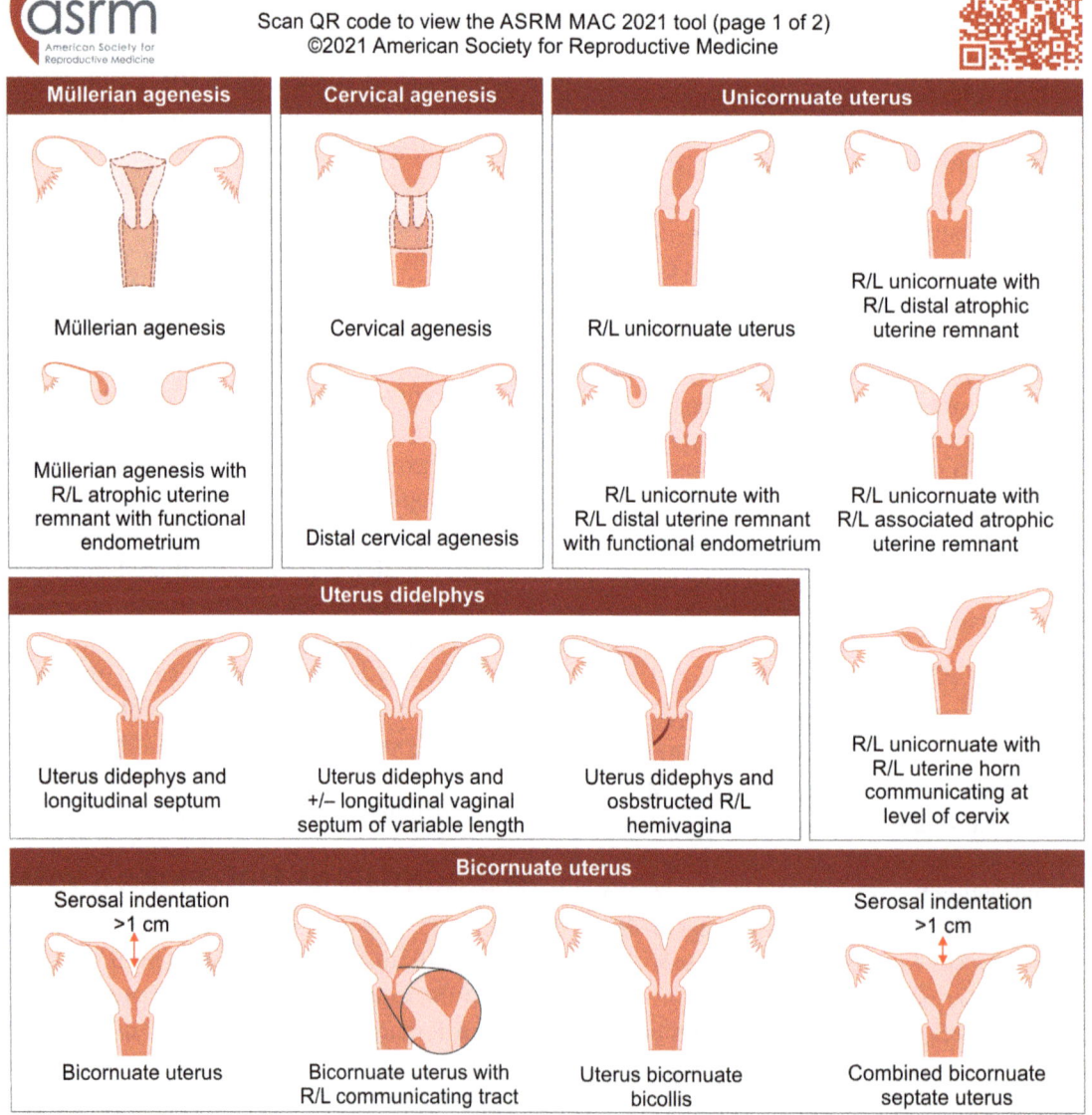

Fig. 1: *Contd...*

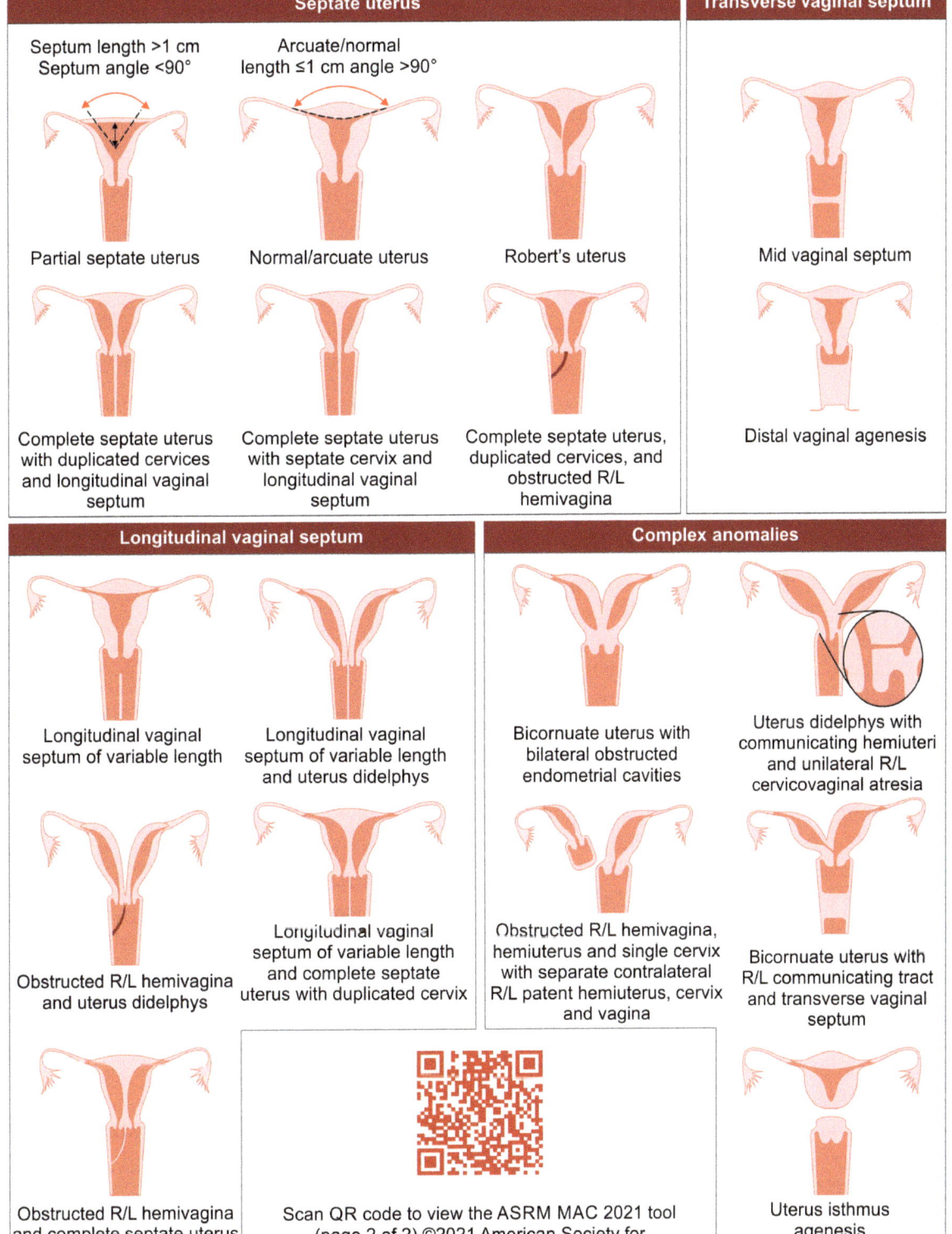

Fig. 1: ASRM classification of Mullerian anomalies. (ASRM: American Society for Reproductive Medicine)

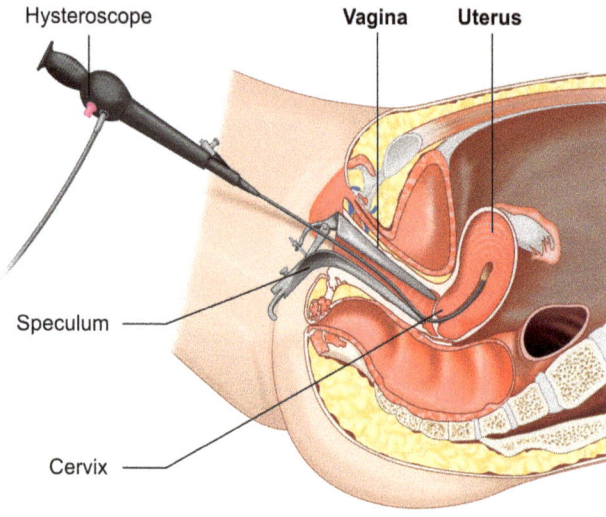

Fig. 2: Hysteroscopy.

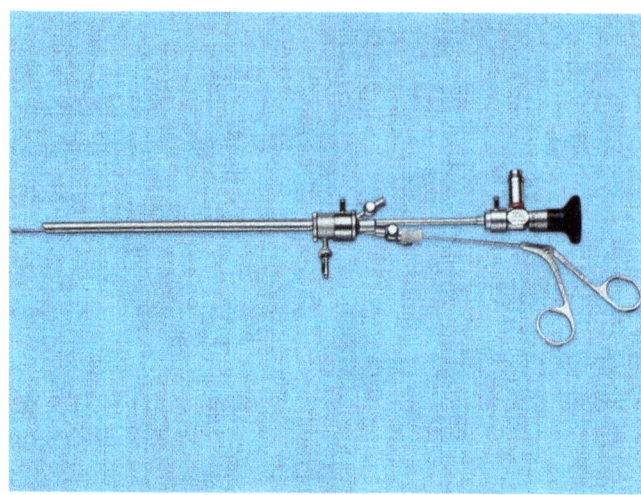

Fig. 3: Hysteroscope with a diameter of 7 mm and a channel for introduction of ancillary instruments.

Hysteroscopic Surgery of Uterine Malformations

Mullerian malformations are a broad category of congenital disorders, mostly affecting young women that are especially related to the reproductive system. Fertility issues are mostly brought on by problems during pregnancy caused by uterine abnormalities. Abortion and early birth are the more typical consequences, occurring in 25% and 16% of patients, respectively. Although it has not been feasible to conclusively demonstrate that uterine malformation is the lone factor causing primary infertility, a number of publications have been published that list a sizable proportion of infertile individuals who also happen to have uterine malformation. Premature births are more common and are linked to didelphic and bicornuate uteri. The majority of pregnancies end at full term without the need for intervention; hence, no therapy is often advised to repair congenital defects. It has been suggested that Strassman metroplasty with subsequent cerclage be used in a few uncommon situations of recurrent abortion. The septate uterus should be surgically treated since it might cause infertility or repeated pregnancy losses.

Instrumentation of Surgical Hysteroscopy

Typically, rigid hysteroscopes with an outer diameter of 7 mm and two channels are used during surgery **(Fig. 3)**. One channel is used to introduce the distension media, and the other is used to introduce ancillary instruments

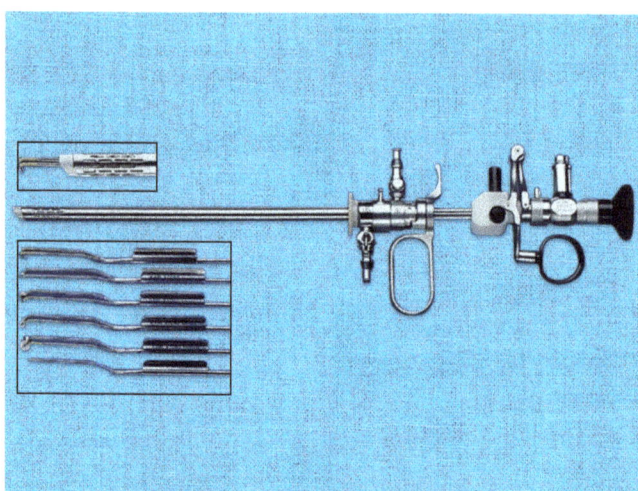

Fig. 4: 26-Fr resectoscope with ancillary electrosurgical instruments.

like probes, catheters, tiny rigid or semi-rigid scissors, and various biopsy forceps **(Figs. 4 and 5)**. A resectoscope is used to perform the majority of hysteroscopic surgery.

Complications of Surgical Hysteroscopy

The liquid distension medium used to enable the visual exploration of the uterine cavity provides the greatest risk in surgical hysteroscopy. The surgeon and anesthesiologist should take the risk of intravasation into account so that they can recognize the syndrome's early symptoms and treat patients as soon as possible.

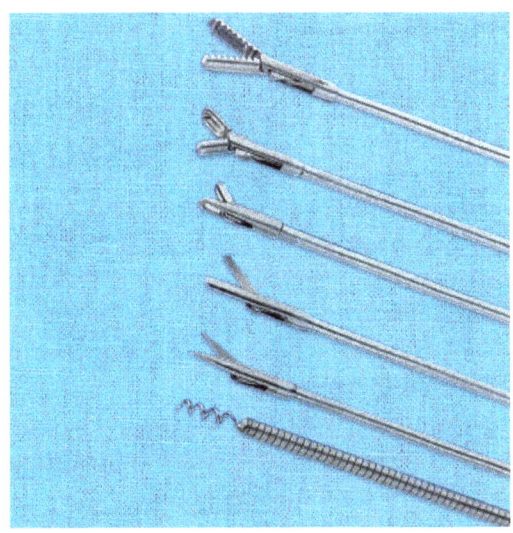

Fig. 5: Instruments used through an operating hysteroscope, forceps, scissors.

Contraindications

There are various contraindications associated with surgical hysteroscopy which includes pelvic inflammatory disease (PID), acute cervicovaginitis, intense menorrhagia, and pregnancy.

HYSTEROSCOPIC APPROACH: PRACTICAL TIPS

The specific role of hysteroscopy in nonseptate MDAs includes:[2]

- *Diagnosis:* Hysteroscopy is a valuable diagnostic tool for identifying nonseptate MDAs. It allows a direct visualization of the uterine cavity and any structural abnormalities within it. This enables healthcare providers to accurately diagnose conditions such as unicornuate uterus, bicornuate uterus, or didelphic uterus.
- *Evaluation of uterine cavity:* Hysteroscopy provides detailed information about the size, shape, and configuration of the uterine cavity. This information is essential for understanding the extent of the anomaly and planning appropriate treatment.
- *Assessment of associated abnormalities:* In addition to identifying the primary uterine anomaly, hysteroscopy can help to detect and assess any associated abnormalities, such as polyps, fibroids, or adhesions, which may contribute to infertility or other gynecological symptoms.
- *Fertility evaluation:* For women with nonseptate MDAs who are experiencing fertility issues, hysteroscopy can be used to assess the impact of the anomaly on fertility. It can help to determine if any surgical correction or assisted reproductive techniques are necessary to improve fertility outcomes.
- *Treatment planning:* In some cases, surgical intervention may be required to correct nonseptate MDAs, especially if they are causing significant symptoms or fertility problems. Hysteroscopy can be used as a minimally invasive surgical approach to correct certain anomalies, such as removing a uterine septum or dividing a bicornuate uterus to create a more normal uterine cavity.
- *Monitoring and follow-up:* After surgical correction or other interventions, hysteroscopy can be used for postoperative evaluation to ensure that the uterine anomaly has been effectively addressed. It can also be utilized for monitoring any potential complications or recurrence of anomalies.
- *Patient counseling:* Hysteroscopy provides visual evidence of the anomaly, which can be used for patient education and counseling. It helps patients to better understand their condition and the treatment options available.

Through hysteroscopy, the uterine cavity and cervical canal may be examined, and the tubal ostium and proximal intramural portion of the fallopian tube can be assessed. The capacity to examine the uterine cavity makes hysteroscopy superior than HSG. Although not always proved by HSG, filling abnormalities and a partial failure of fusion of the Mullerian ducts might be suspected.[8]

Entry: The preferred route of entry into the uterine cavity is by using the vaginoscopy- hysteroscopy technique. This ensures that the entire vagina, its fornices, and the cervical anatomy, along with the external os are clearly visualized before an entry is made into the cavity. This ensures that even minor defects are not missed out. Some of the anomalies/abnormalities that could be detected at this stage are:[8]

- *Complete vaginal septum—associated with a complete uterine + cervical septum:* Both halves of the vagina and both hemicervices are inspected after distending each hemi vagina with the distension medium. The telescope is inserted in each hemi cavity and both ostia visualized.

- *Transverse vaginal septum*—possibly associated with agenesis of the lower cervix/upper vagina. A pinpoint opening of the transverse septum may be seen, though in most cases it is too small to be negotiated with a telescope. Anomalies of the vaginal septum should be resected at the time of diagnosis, thereby resolving problems of dyspareunia and permitting adequate drainage of menstrual flow.
- Concomitant puckering and nodularity of the posterior fornix suggesting rectovaginal septum endometriosis—frequently associated with a noncommunicating functional hemi uterus and pelvic endometriosis.
- A pinpoint external os—in patients with hypoplastic uterus
- Cervix completely flushed to the vaginal wall

Patients who have a cervical agenesis diagnosis should be referred for a hysterectomy, which should preferably be done laparoscopically. Many surgical attempts to construct a cervix have ended tragically, frequently due to deadly consequences. In view of the obstetrical problems, the chances of conception with in vitro fertilization techniques should be assessed, and these women should be given possible alternatives. In such circumstances, using a surrogate womb might be the best choice.[9]

The view from the internal os: Once the internal os has been negotiated, the first look into the cavity provides a wealth of information. The surgeon must carefully inspect the fundus, lateral walls, and both ostial openings from the vantage point of the internal os. On inspection, a "normal" uterus should have the following features **(Fig. 6)**.

- The fundus is usually curved slightly inward, rather than completely flat. Subsequently, the area between the two ostia appears slightly elevated and projecting into the cavity.
- The two ostia are equidistant from the midline.
- Both ostia are seen in one single view (not a very consistent finding).
- If the two ostia are not seen together in a single frame, each ostium is at least visible from the internal os when the light cable is tilted from the 6 o'clock to the 3 and 9 o'clock positions.
- The overall cavity appears "spacious". This is a subjective assessment, learnt over a period of time after performing a number of cases.

Any variations to this anatomy should raise the suspicion of a uterine anomaly. Of course, the hysteroscopy findings must complement, and not dispute the diagnosis that has been made on imaging preoperatively.

- *The T-shaped uterus:* Beyond the internal os, a tubular, tunnel-like hollow can be observed. None of the tubal ostia can be visualized. The telescope needs to be inserted farther into the uterine cavity, typically past the halfway point. At this point, visualizing the tubal ostium is made possible by tilting the light wire. The view of just one of the ostia may be obstructed by the hypertrophied lateral wall in the case of a unilaterally convergent wall (the 7-shaped uterus), while the other ostium is plainly visible from the internal os **(Fig. 7)**.

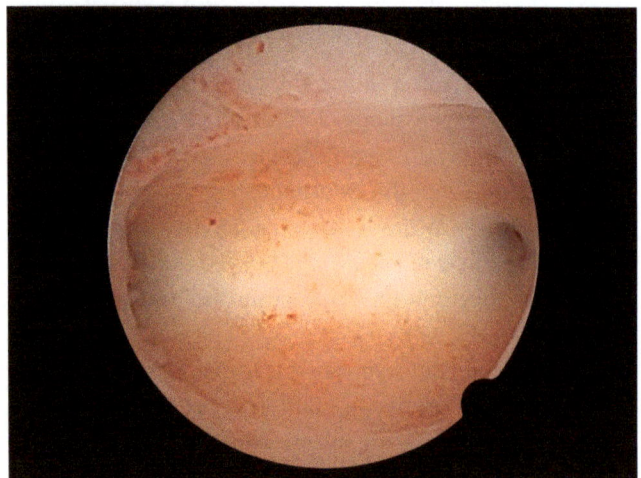

Fig. 6: Normal uterine cavity.

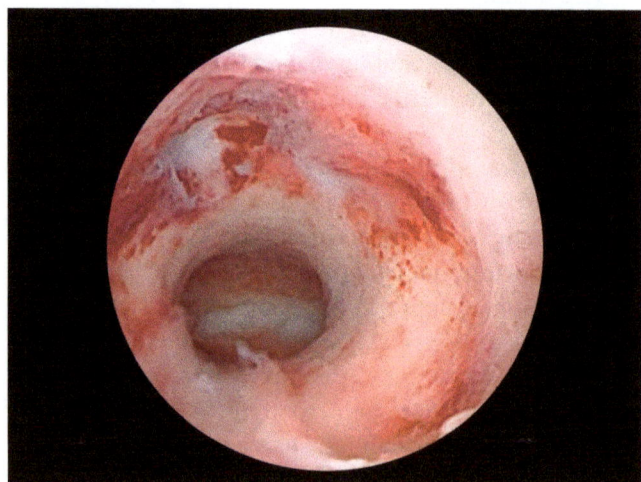

Fig. 7: Narrow cavity of T-shaped uterus.

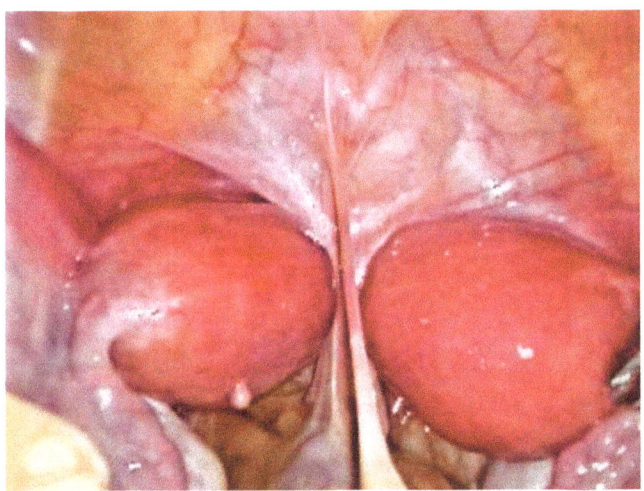

Fig. 8: Laparoscopic view of bicornuate uterus.

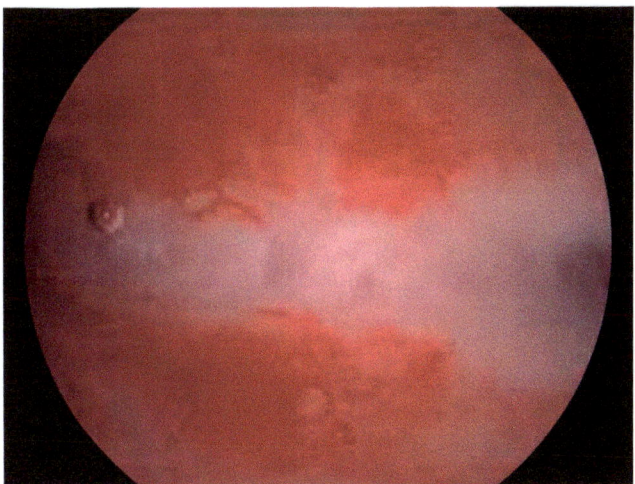

Fig. 9: Hysteroscopic view of unicornuate uterus.

- Making this observation carefully at this stage is very important, because this is also considered as the end point of surgical correction once the lateral wall has been incised with an electrode or a scissor.
- *The bicornuate uterus*: The cavity of a bicornuate unicollis uterus has the exact same appearance as a uterus that is entirely septated. It is crucial to distinguish between the two because if the uterus is bicornuate, or bicorporeal septate, rather than septate, a careless septal incision started by simply observing an inward midline depression might result in a catastrophic perforation. This distinction can be determined either intraoperatively by doing a concurrent diagnostic laparoscopy or preoperatively by employing a 3D ultrasound to determine the degree of serosal indentation **(Fig. 8)**.
- *The unicornuate uterus:* With a single terminal ostium, a banana-shaped cavity is observed as opposed to a tubular one. The cavity's volume is obviously less. The surgeon must be careful to avoid mistakenly visualizing only one-half of a bicornuate uterus and mislabeling it as a unicornuate uterus by failing to see the other half. It is advisable to undergo a concurrent diagnostic laparoscopy to determine the second horn's dimensions and functions **(Fig. 9)**.

  Laparoscopy should be used to excise obstructed, rudimentary uterine horns, and adjacent tubes in patients with a unicornuate uterus.[9]
- *Accessory cavitated uterine mass (ACUM)*: Previously known as juvenile cystic adenoma (JCA), ultrasound leaves behind a diagnostic dilemma, confusing the entity with a functional noncommunicating uterine horn with hematometra. In both cases, the patient presents with severe dysmenorrhea. In these cases, a diagnostic hysteroscopy performed before laparoscopy effectively rules out the possibility of a noncommunicating horn, if both ostia are visualized **(Figs. 10A to C)**.[10]

  Accessory cavitated uterine mass is a difficult condition to diagnose. One needs a high index of suspicion. Since most patients with ACUM suffer from dysmenorrhea, surgical excision is necessary and can be easily done by laparoscopy. When a cystic lesion seen in the myometrium is asymptomatic, it is difficult to distinguish ACUM from its differential diagnoses and a correct diagnosis can be made only after excision and histopathological evaluation.
- *The Robert's uterus:* This condition is also best diagnosed by preoperative pelvic MRI, and is an asymmetric fusion of the vaginal septum to one side of the midline **(Fig. 11)**. Consequently, hematocolpos and hematometra, sometimes hematosalpinx ensues. On vaginoscopy, a bulge is seen distending one-half of the vagina, and only half the circumference of the cervix is visible. The appearance of the uterine cavity, before corrective surgery is performed, is like a unicornuate uterus.[11]

  Laparoscopy should also be used for hysterectomy in cases of cervical agenesis and in neovaginoplasty procedures in cases of vaginal agenesis **(Figs. 12A and B)**.

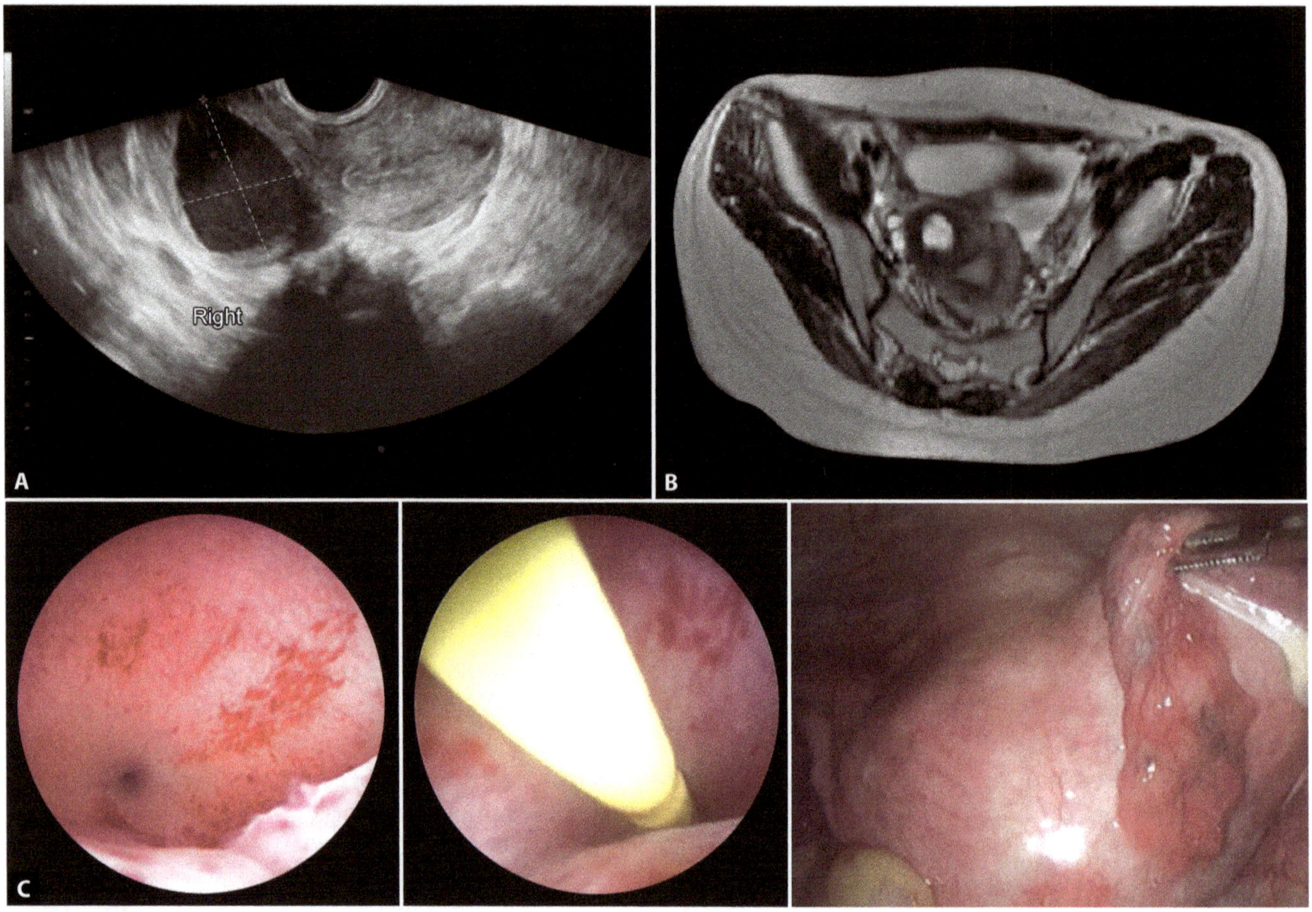

Figs. 10A to C: (A) Transrectal ultrasonography shows a cystic lesion on the right cornual part of the uterus; (B) MRI shows a cystic lesion on the right side of the uterus. There was no communication between the endometrial cavity and the cystic lesion; (C) Showing hysteroscopic cannulation of the right tubal ostium and chromopertubation showing that the right tube is patent.

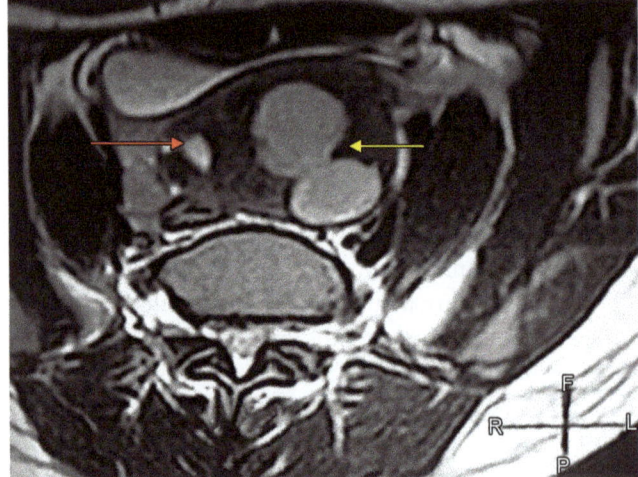

Fig. 11: Magnetic resonance imaging of pelvis showing uterine septum dividing endometrial cavity asymmetrically into normal right side uterine cavity (red arrow) and left side (yellow arrow) noncommunicating uterine cavity.

In many women, the malformation results in obstructed and retrograde menstruation, thereby facilitating the development of endometriosis **(Figs. 13A and B)**. During laparoscopy, this diagnosis may be confirmed and the endometrial foci may be resected **(Figs. 14A to C)**.

CONCLUSION

The MDAs are embryologic anomalies that may be associated with congenital urinary tract or cervicothoracic somite anomalies that may vary from person to person. It is important to note that the specific management of non-septate MDAs will depend on the individual patient's clinical presentation, reproductive goals, and the severity of the anomaly. Therefore, the role of hysteroscopy may vary from case to case, and decisions should be made in consultation with a gynecologist or reproductive specialist who has expertise in managing these conditions.

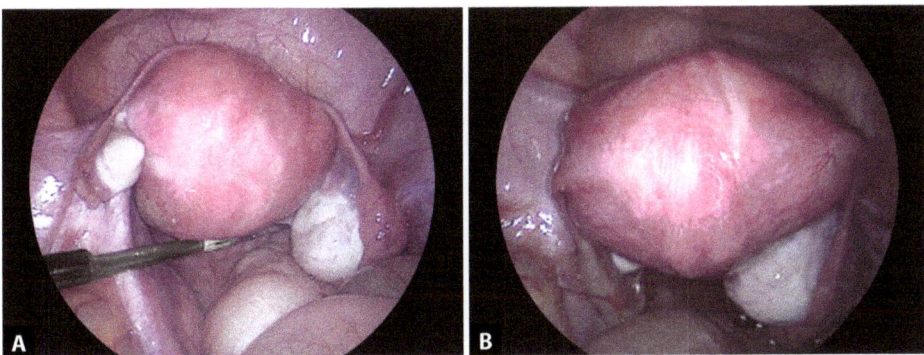

Figs. 12A and B: (A) Laparoscopic findings pre-excision of uterine septum. Bulge is seen on the left side of fundus due to hematometra on the left side of uterine cavity; (B) Postoperative laparoscopic view of normal fundus after excision of uterine septum.

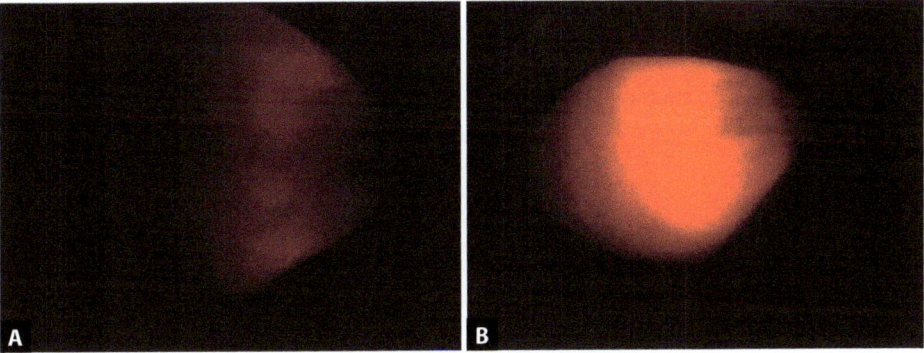

Figs. 13A and B: (A) Hysteroscopic illumination of uterine cavity; right half of cavity is illuminated as left side is obliterated due to hematometra; (B) Postexcision of uterine septum entire uterine cavity is illuminated.

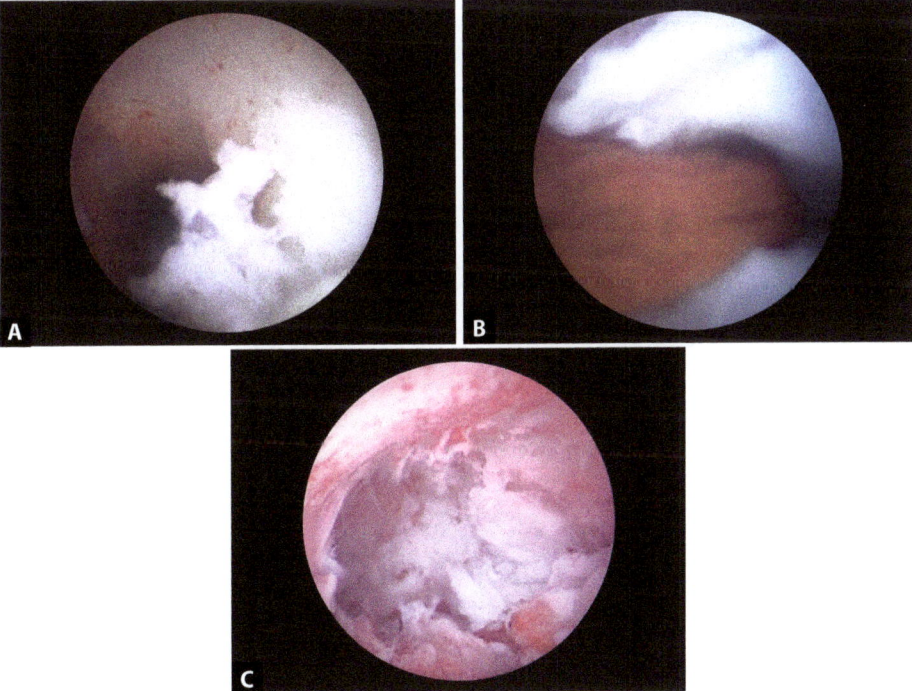

Figs. 14A to C: (A) On hysteroscopy, right side cavity and ostium are visualized and left-sided septal bulge is seen due to asymmetric uterine septum; (B) Uterine septum is excised using scissors. Left side hematometra is drained; (C) Hysteroscopic view of unified endometrial cavity after septal resection.

REFERENCES

1. Sugi MD, Penna R, Jha P, Pōder L, Behr SC, Courtier J, et al. Müllerian duct anomalies: Role in Fertility and Pregnancy. Radiographics. 2021;41(6):1857-75.
2. Buttram VC Jr. Müllerian anomalies and their management. Fertil Steril. 1983;40(2):159-63.
3. Chandler TM, Machan LS, Cooperberg PL, Harris AC, Chang SD. Mullerian duct anomalies: from diagnosis to intervention. Br J Radiol. 2009;82(984):1034-42.
4. Bhagavath B, Ellie G, Griffiths KM, Winter T, Alur-Gupta S, Richardson C, et al. Uterine malformations: an update of diagnosis, Management, and Outcomes. Obstet Gynecol Surv. 2017;72(6):377-92.
5. Pfeifer SM, Attaran M, Goldstein J, Lindheim SR, Petrozza JC, Rackow BW, et al. ASRM müllerian anomalies classification 2021. Fertil Steril. 2021;116(5):1238-52.
6. Ludwin A, Pfeifer SM. Reproductive surgery for müllerian anomalies: a review of progress in the last decade. Fertil Steril. 2019;112(3):408-16.
7. Saravelos SH, Cocksedge KA, Li TC. Prevalence and diagnosis of congenital uterine anomalies in women with reproductive failure: a critical appraisal. Hum Reprod Update. 2008;14(5):415-29.
8. Pisat S. (2023). Diagnostic hysteroscopy for congenital anomalies of the female genital system – ISGE. [online] Available from: https://www.isge.org/2023/04/diagnostic-hysteroscopy-for-congenital-anomalies-of-the-female-genital-system/#:~:text=Hysteroscopic%20approach&text=This%20ensures%20that%20the%20entire,defects%20are%20not%20missed%20out. [Last accessed November, 2023].
9. Ribeiro SC, Tormena RA, Peterson TV, Gonzáles Mde O, Serrano PG, Almeida JA, et al. Müllerian duct anomalies: review of current management. Sao Paulo Med J. 2009;127(2):92-6.
10. Supermaniam S, Thye WL. Diagnosis and laparoscopic excision of accessory cavitated uterine mass in young women: Two case reports. Case Rep Womens Health. 2020;26:e00187.
11. Shah N, Changede P. Hysteroscopic management of Robert's uterus. J Obstet Gynaecol India. 2020;70(1):86-8.

Chapter 8: Intrauterine Adhesions: Systematic Approach

S Krishnakumar, Shrutika O Makde

■ INTRODUCTION

Intrauterine adhesions (IUAs) coined after Asherman, 1948, was initially described by Fritsch, 1894.[1] From Asherman's original definition, the syndrome was a consequence of trauma to the endometrium, producing partial or complete obliteration in the uterine cavity and/or the cervical canal, resulting in conditions such as menstrual abnormalities, infertility, and recurrent pregnancy loss.[2] "Asherman's" term denotes a condition with varying symptoms, manifestations, and pathology, there cannot be one single definition of Asherman's syndrome (AS) with strict inclusion and exclusion criteria and indicating an endometrial disorder of great significance, one with important reproductive consequences and other.[1]

■ TYPES AND ETIOLOGY

Endometrium undergoes cyclical changes with growth and sloughing every month and the pathology for this layer to get adherent is poorly understood.[3] Prevalence varies from 0.3 to 21.5%.[2,4] Adhesions are composed of fibrotic tissue resulting in the adherence of opposing surfaces. It is possible that, after injury to the endometrium, fibrosis may follow with the potential for adhesion formation **(Table 1)**.[2] Etiological determinants of Asherman's syndrome are trauma to the uterine cavity by curettage (especially puerperal uterus), local infection, or a combination of these factors.[3,5] Shokeir et al., 2008, found 6.7% of patients undergoing hysteroscopic septal resection to have IUAs.[6]

Although endometritis is said to be a predisposing factor, most with IUA have had no clinical evidence

TABLE 1: ASRM classification of intrauterine adhesions.

The American Fertility Society classification of intrauterine adhesions, 1988:

Extent of cavity involved	<1/3	1/3–2/3	>2/3
	1	2	4
Type of adhesions	Filmy	Filmy and dense	Dense
	1	2	4
Menstrual pattern	Normal	Hypomenorrhea	Amenorrhea
	0	2	4
Prognostic classification		**HSG[a] score**	**Hysteroscopy score**
Stage I		(Mild)	1–4
Stage II		(Moderate)	5–8
Stage III		(Severe)	9–12

[a]All adhesions should be considered dense.
Yu D, Wong YM, Cheong Y, Xia E, Li TC. Asherman syndrome—one century later. Fertil Steril. 2008;89(4): 759-79.
(ASRM: American Society for Reproductive Medicine; HSG: hysterosalpingography)
Source: American Fertility Society. The American Fertility Society classifications of adnexal adhesions, distal tubal occlusion, tubal occlusion secondary to tubal ligation, tubal pregnancies, mullerian anomalies and intrauterine adhesions. Fertil Steril. 1988;49:944-55.

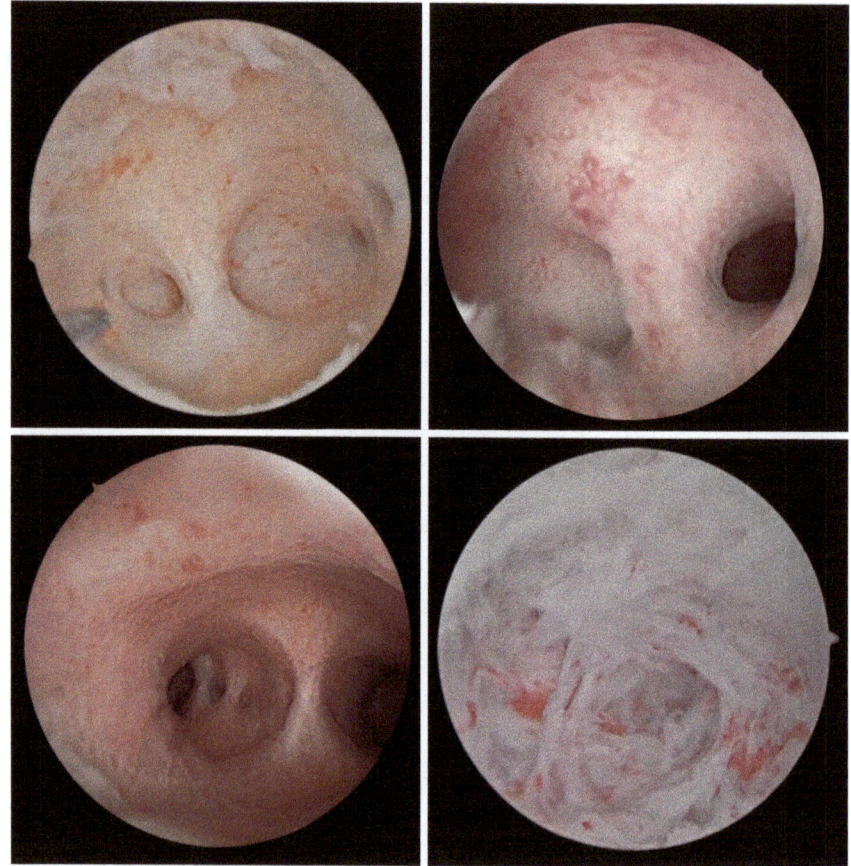

Fig. 1: Various stages intrauterine adhesions—mild, moderate, and severe.

of infection, except for tubercle bacillus which causes extensive endometrial destruction in absence of uterine surgery.[7]

Stillman and Asarkof (1985) found Mullerian anomalies in 8.0% and AS in 4.8%, though no data proves that anomalous uteri are more prone to develop IUA after curettage than is a normal uterus.[8]

■ DIAGNOSIS

Several diagnostic modalities have been used for evaluation of IUA. Difficulty to sound the uterus should raise suspicion of presence of IUA. Transvaginal sonography can assess endometrial development, can identify areas of calcification as well as hyperechoic areas which correlate with dense adhesions and may detect a hematometra.[3] Hysterosalpingography (HSG) gives the opportunity to simultaneously evaluate tubal patency, but details of filling defects are not visualized, and a high false-positive rate is documented.[9] If uterine sounding fails, instead of HSG or saline infusion sonogram (SIS), hysteroscopy must be done as, if a sound will not pass, neither will iodine contrast nor saline. Difficulties in diagnosing IUAs were solved by the introduction of hysteroscopy, which is the gold standard modality **(Fig. 1)**.[3,9]

Virtual hysteroscopy, a 4D virtual reconstruction of the uterine cavity may play a future role in the diagnosis of IUA.[10] In these rare cases, MRI can be valuable, although too expensive as a routine diagnostic too.[11]

The diagnosis of AS should be based on:
- At least one of the clinical features including amenorrhea, subfertility, hypomenorrhea, recurrent pregnancy loss, or history related to abnormal placentation including previa and accreta.
- The presence of IUAs by hysteroscopy and/or histologically confirmed intrauterine fibrosis.[2]

■ PLANNING

Surgery is the only treatment modality available in symptomatic IUAs. There are no randomized control trials of any treatment versus expectant management or any other treatment.

The objective of treatment is:
- To restore the shape and volume of the uterine cavity to normal
- To facilitate communication between the cavity and both the cervical canal and the fallopian tubes.

Treat associated symptoms including infertility and prevent recurrence of adhesions.

Hysteroscopic treatment has become the method of choice as it can be performed under vision with minimal trauma. However, future fertility treatment may be necessary, especially in case where the tubes are blocked.[9]

OPERATIVE TIPS

With increasing application of miniature hysteroscopes (2.9 mm, 2.7 mm, and 1.9 mm) with overall diameter of operative sheath reduced to 3.5 mm, even in very difficult cases of cervical stenosis and adhesions, it is easy to negotiate and complete a good job inside the uterine cavity. Today we can plan before beginning of any hysteroscopic surgery whether one has to use operative hysteroscopy or resectoscopic surgery **(Fig. 2)**.

It is imperative that one adapts the vaginoscopic approach for hysteroscopy as one can appreciate all adhesions right from the cervical canal and negotiate the cervical canal under vision. It is important to perform first a complete diagnostic evaluation of the cervical canal and uterine cavity to familiarize with the anatomical landmarks inside the uterine cavity, before embarking upon any adhesiolysis. Also, one has to remember that intrauterine adhesiolysis should be attempted, by an experienced hysteroscopic surgeon. Adhesiolysis usually begins inferiorly and can be advanced cephalically until the uterine architecture has been normalized.

Which instrument and when?

Adhesiolysis can be performed through operative hysteroscopy by using:
- Hysteroscopic scissors (5 Fr and 7 Fr) **(Fig. 3)**
- Bipolar needle

Adhesions in the cervical canal and at the level of internal os can be many a time negotiated by just opening the blades of the scissors and only use the blades for cutting if the adhesions cannot be negotiated. Filmy adhesion can be dissected by using the tip of the hysteroscope without any energy source or scissors. Filmy and central adhesions should be divided first as these are more easily distinguished; marginal and dense adhesions are more difficult to identify, and divisions of

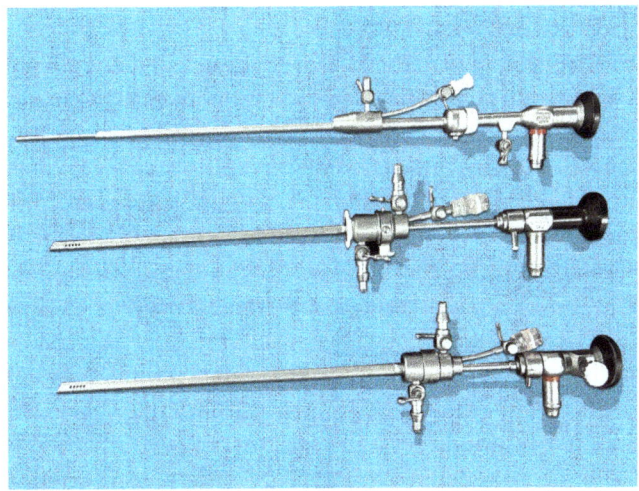

Fig. 2: Operative hysteroscopic sheaths of increasing size—4 mm, 5 mm, and 7 mm operative.

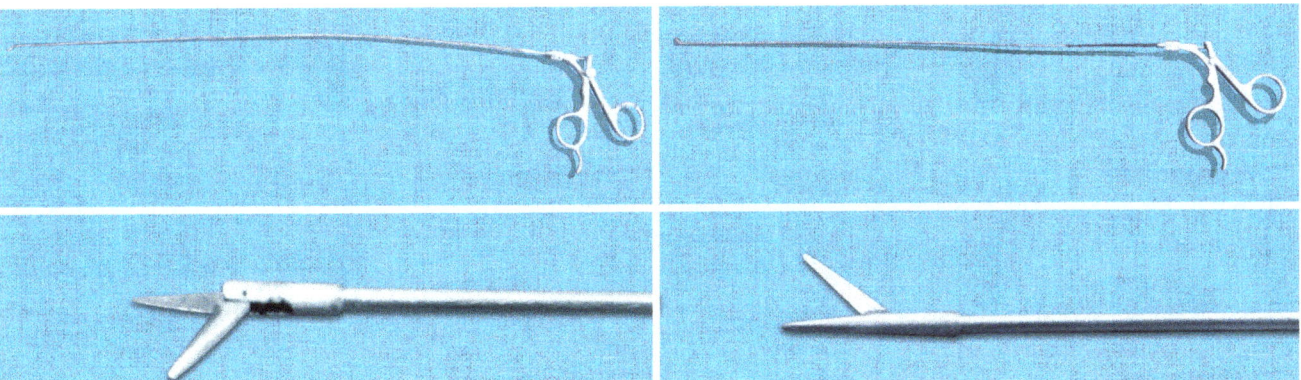

Fig. 3: Pointed scissors with figure showing operative end.

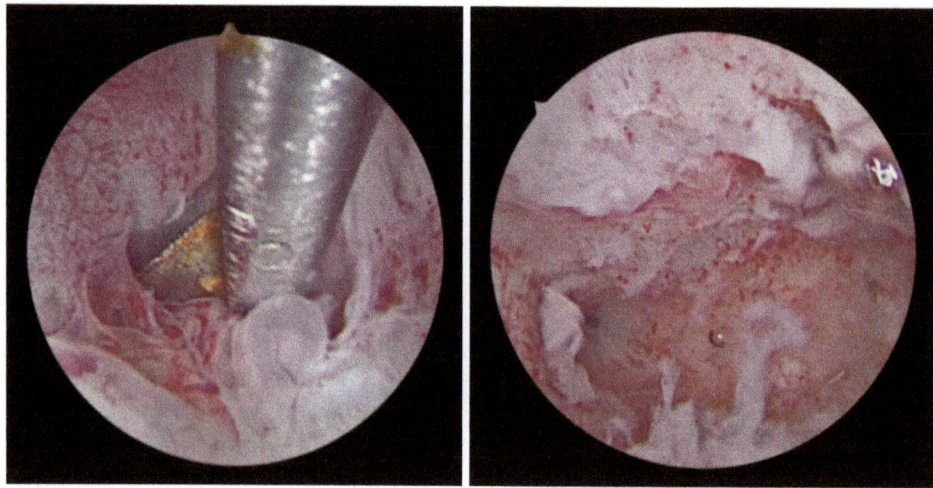

Fig. 4: Hysteroscopic adhesiolysis with scissors in case of intrauterine adhesions and the postoperative image.

these adhesions, sometimes may be difficult to manage with scissors.

The cases where the internal os is also obliterated and one may not be able to enter the endometrial cavity. In this situation, one must remember that the cervical mucosal folds lining the whole circumference of the cervical canal will converge at the anatomical internal os. Hence, one must follow to the converging point and there gradually start cutting with sharp scissors or can rotate the scissors and open the blade and dilate the internal os **(Fig. 4)**.

The main advantage of using scissors for adhesiolysis is that use of "no energy" minimizes the inadvertent damage to the residual endometrium. Over the years with experience, we prefer to use scissors only in all cases of Asherman's and in the last 10 years never ever resorted to any energy.

If use of energy is desired in some cases then bipolar needles are excellent tools as they can be used to achieve precise cutting and good hemostasis.[12] Another advantage of bipolar needle is one can use normal saline, since it is a bipolar modality. But the main disadvantage of the electrodes is that they are very delicate and does not last for many cases, adding to the cost **(Fig. 5)**.

Whenever, it is not possible to lyse the adhesions with scissors or bipolar needle, one can opt for resectoscopic surgery with Collins knife. Resectoscope if required, the bipolar mini resectoscope should be used where blind dilatation is not needed as in case of Global AS the risk of creation of blind passage is high.

Whenever thermal energy is used to divide adhesions, minimum amount of energy must be used to avoid

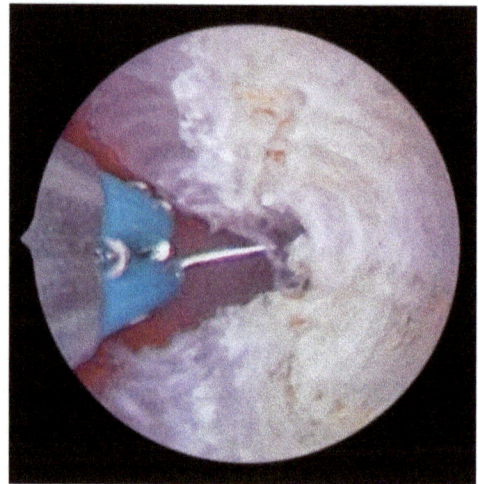

Fig. 5: Bipolar needle in mini resectoscope.

further damage of endometrial tissue. Whenever one is using energy for adhesiolysis, all safety guidelines for hysteroscopic surgery should be followed and one should always keep the tubal ostia under vision.

In some instances, even after extensive hysteroscopic adhesiolysis, intrauterine landmarks remain obscure; and one should not continue the adhesiolysis just to see the tubal ostia in these cases. One must stop the procedure if adequate uterine cavity size and shape is created and in second look hysteroscopy one may see the tubal ostia clearly, though it may not be seen in the first sitting.

Hysteroscopic diode lasers—the diode laser with a fiber of 1,470 nm can also be used for adhesiolysis but as mentioned avoid energy sources as far as possible and use mechanical methods such as scissors.

Assisted guidance—hysteroscopic adhesiolysis: Fluoroscopic guidance using a Tuohy needle has been used to guide pockets of endometrium have been described,[13] but there are no long-term data for this technique, and seem to be limited for mild adhesions only.

The USG (transabdominal, transrectal) guided hysteroscopic adhesiolysis has been reported to reduce the risk of uterine perforation.[14] However, since all the studies are small, and success and perforation prevention is both surgeon and sonographer-dependent, its use cannot be recommended without further research.

The use of laparoscopic guidance is controversial because, although its use has been suggested during division of severe IUAs, perforations have been reported.[15] Laparoscopy during hysteroscopy is best considered for immediate recognition and treatment during accidental perforation with intrauterine adhesiolysis.

Readhesion prevention strategies: The postoperative strategies to prevent IUA include barriers (physical/gel) to separate the opposing walls and regenerate the endometrium faster.

- *Physical barriers*:
  - *Intrauterine devices (IUD)*: IUD was the first physical barrier between the uterine walls,[16] to be used after adhesiolysis, but is no longer recommended as Lippe's loop, once considered IUD of choice after adhesiolysis is no longer available, and copper containing IUDs provoke inflammatory reaction, and also T-shaped IUDs have too small a surface area to be truly effective to act as a physical barrier. Also the risk of infection into the uterus was quantified as 8% in one series.
  - *Intrauterine balloon stent*: An intrauterine balloon stent made of silicone, which because of its triangular shape conforms to the configuration of a normal uterus and maintains separation at the margins of the uterine cavity, which is where reformation is common, is placed immediately after completing adhesiolysis. In a large trial of 1,240 patients treated using intrauterine stent, pregnancy rate of 61.6% and spontaneous miscarriage rate of 15.6%. No data about IUA recurrence has been reported. In an RCT comparing the efficacy of intrauterine balloon and intrauterine device in prevention of adhesion reformation, it was found that there was no significant difference in the incidence and the amount of adhesion reformation between the IUD group and intrauterine balloon group[17] **(Fig. 6)**.

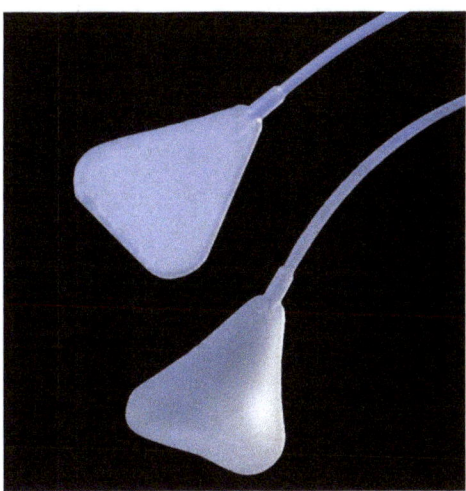

Fig. 6: Intrauterine balloon stent.

  - *Pediatric Foley catheter:* A no. 8 or 10 Foley catheter, with 3 mL distension of its bulb for 3–10 days after lysis of IUAs, has been reported in several studies, with good results like the balloon stent with much reduced cost. We routinely cut the tip of the catheter, to fit the bulb, properly close to fundus. In a retrospective study conducted by Ru Zhu, Hua Duan et al., it was concluded that recurrence rate of postoperative adhesions was less in ISB group than that of FB group (25% *vs.* 35.1%). The difference was seen more in severe Asherman's group and was attributed mainly to the uterine cavity drainage catheter of the ISB which can drain the exudate early after the operation and reduce the formation of adhesions. The adhesion in the FB group were seen more in the periphery and top of the uterine cavity as the separation of the walls may be less with Foley balloon in these areas.[18] Use of fresh amnion graft over an inflated Foley catheter has also been used with encouraging results1 **(Fig. 7)**.

In a systemic review, Di Spiezo Sardo et al. (2016) have concluded that Foley catheter is better than IUD, but inferior to balloon stent. Amnion graft, especially if fresh, seems to improve the results of other physical barriers.

- *Gel barriers*

Hyaluronic acid and adhesion barriers: Hyaluronic acid generates a temporary barrier between organs,

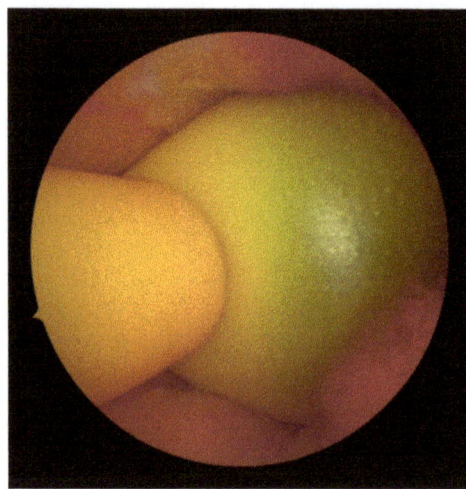

Fig. 7: Pediatric Foleys bulb in situ.

preventing adhesion formation and also is known to influence tissue repair by proliferation of mesothelial cells. An initial hyaluronic acid–based product, ferric hyaluronic acid, was removed from market because of its toxicity.

- Auto-cross-linked hyaluronic acid gel (Hyalobarrier gel) may be more suitable to prevent IUAs. In a prospective randomized control trial of 84 women, this gel was compared with no therapy after adhesiolysis, hysteroscopically which showed that the walls of the uterine cavity remained separated for at least 72 hours. At second look hysteroscopy 3 months after the surgery, IUAs were significantly reduced in patients receiving the adhesion barrier (14%), compared with the control (32%).[19]
- Seprafilm, a chemically modified hyaluronic acid and carboxymethylcellulose combination, has also been tried with encouraging results in several studies. A brand new hyaluronic acid (alginate carboxymethylcellulose hyaluronic acid) was evaluated in a prospective randomized trial including 187 cases.[20] 4 weeks after surgery, IUAs were significantly lower compared with carboxymethylcellulose hyaluronic acid.
- Oxiplex/AP Gel (Fzio Med, INC San Luis Obispo, CA), a formulation of viscoelastic gel, was shown in preclinical studies to be most effective in reducing adhesions to peritoneal surfaces following surgery. It is a sterile nonpyrogenic gel adjusted to isotonicity with sodium chloride. It is a new intraperitoneal gelatinous compound that is composed of polyethylene oxide and carboxymethyl cellulose stabilized by calcium chloride. Carboxymethyl cellulose decreases the injured tissue apposition required for adhesion formation.

A high number of randomized and nonrandomized studies have shown that intrauterine application of antiadhesive gel is an effective strategy for preventing postoperative IUA.

- *Hormone therapy:* Hormone therapy typically is given in cases where one would want the endometrium to grow and epithelialize the raw surface as in cases of septal incision, Asherman adhesiolysis, and never in cases of fibroid or polyp resection. In 1964, Wood and Pena described estrogen therapy to stimulate regeneration of the endometrium after intrauterine adhesiolysis.[21] Healing after septoplasty was reported to be the slowest of intrauterine procedures compared with myomectomy and polypectomy with the highest rate of de novo adhesions formation occurring in 148 of 169 (88%) women compared with 26 of 65 (40%) after myomectomy and 0 of 37 after polypectomy (43%). Surprisingly most studies after septoplasty have shown no benefit in terms of preventing adhesion or subsequent pregnancy rates in patients receiving adhesion barriers and hormonal treatment when compared to women undergoing septoplasty where none was used.

Since then, various regimens have been described, but no comparative studies have been performed on dosage, administration, or combination of hormones. The most popular is the use of conjugated equine estrogen in a daily dose of 2.5 mg for 20 days followed by progesterone for 5 days for two to three cycles. Estradiol valerate at a dose of 4 mg per day can also be used in place of Premarin.[22] Preoperative estrogen therapy has also been suggested to be of potential benefit in increasing endometrial thickness before any surgical intervention, although data are limited. The role of hormonal therapy is difficult to evaluate as most studies have included hormonal treatment in addition to other treatment strategies. Adverse effects of estrogen and progesterone must be evaluated in the absence of evidence, with nausea, headache, and the risk of thromboembolic disease considered if using this treatment.

- *Drugs to increase vascular flow to endometrium:* Various drugs such as aspirin, nitroglycerine, and sildenafil citrate have been used in various case reports to

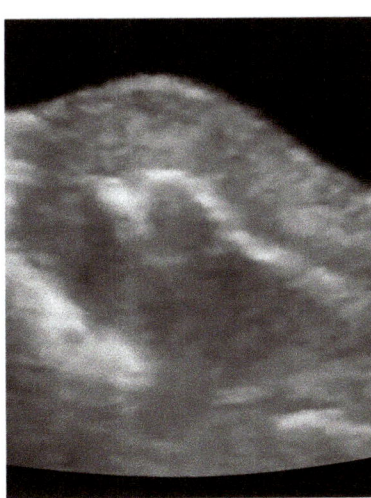

Fig. 8: Use of intermittent balloon dilatation to under ultrasonography guidance.

increase vascular perfusion to endometrium. Though, their results have been encouraging in isolated cases, at this time, they cannot be recommended as an ancillary treatment after lysis of IUAs.
- *Stem cell and endometrial regeneration:* There is substantial evidence in literature that adult endometrial tissue contains epithelial progenitor cells and mesenchymal/stromal (MSC) cells. These cells could be the target of a specific therapy in order to regenerate the endometrial tissue in cases of dysfunctional or atrophic endometrium in future. Bone marrow stem cells contribute for endometrium regeneration. Woman with severe AS treated with autologous bone marrow derived stem cells from endometrial regeneration led to a successful implantation.

A novel technique as described by X Shi et al. is intermittent balloon dilatation therapy on 2 week and 6 weeks following adhesiolysis, is cheap, feasible, and effective, and has been suggested in order to decrease the adhesions reformation rate with significant results (Fig. 8).

CONCLUSION

- Intrauterine adhesions cause significant impact on the reproductive life of woman.
- Hysteroscopy is the gold standard modality to diagnose and treat IUA.
- The division of adhesions begins in the central and safe part of the uterus and moves laterally and toward the fundus.
- Avoid use of energy sources for adhesiolysis to decrease the rates of complication and minimize destruction of endometrium.
- Readhesion prevention strategies are equally important to prevent recurrence of IUA.

REFERENCES

1. March CM. Management of Asherman's syndrome. Reprod Biomed Online. 2011;23(1):63-76.
2. Yu D, Wong YM, Cheong Y, Xia E, Li TC. Asherman syndrome—one century later. Fertil Steril. 2008;89(4): 759-79.
3. Westendorp IC, Ankum WM, Mol BW, Vonk J. Prevalence of Asherman's syndrome after secondary removal of placental remnants or a repeat curettage for incomplete abortion. Hum Reprod. 1998;13(12):3347-50.
4. Schenker JG, Margalioth EJ. Intrauterine adhesions: an updated appraisal. Fertil Steril. 1982;37:593-610.
5. Rabau E, David A. Intrauterine adhesions, etiology, prevention, and treatment. Obstet Gynecol. 1963;22(5):626-9.
6. Shokeir TA, Fawzy M, Tatungy M. The nature of intrauterine adhesions following reproductive hysteroscopic surgery as determined by early and late follow-up hysteroscopy: clinical implications. Acta Gynecol Obstet. 2008;277: 423-7.
7. Polishuk WZ, Anteby SO, Weinstein D. Puerperal endometritis and intrauterine adhesions. Int Surg. 1975;60:418-20.
8. Stillman RJ, Asarkof N. Association between mullerian duct malformation and Asherman syndrome in infertile women. Obstet Gynecol. 1985;65:673-7.
9. Dreisler E, Kjer JJ. Asherman's syndrome: Current perspectives on diagnosis and management. Int J Womens Health. 2019;11:191-8.
10. Tesarik J, Mendoza-Tesarik R, Mendoza N. Virtual ultrasonographic hysteroscopy followed by conventional operative hysteroscopy, enabling pregnancy. Am J Obstet Gynecol. 2017;216(2):188.e1.
11. Bacelar AC, Wilcock D, Powell M, Worthington BS. The value of MRI in the assessment of traumatic intrauterine adhesions (Asherman's syndrome). Clin Radiol. 1995;50(2):80-3.
12. Protopapas A, Shushan A, Magos A. Mymetrial scoring: a new technique for the management of severe Asheman's Syndrome. Fertil Steril. 1998;69:860-4.
13. Valle RF, Sciarra J. Intrauterine adhesions: Hysteroscopic diagnosis, classification, treatment, and reproductive outcome. Am J Obstet Gynecol. 1988;158:1459-70.
14. Broome JD, Vancaille T. Fleuoroscopically guided hysteroscopic division of adhesions in severe Asherman syndrome. Obstet Gynecol. 1999;6:1041-3.
15. Bellingham FR. Intrauterine adhesions: hysteroscopic lysis and adjunctive methods. Aust N Z J Obstet Gynecol. 1996;36:171-4.

16. Di Spiezio Sardo A, Bettochi S, Spinelli M, Guida M, Nappi L, Angioni S, et al. Review of new office-based hysteroscopic procedures 2003-2009. J Minim Invasive Gynecol. 2010;17:436-48.
17. Bettochi S, Nappi Z, Ceci O, Selvaggi L. Office hysteroscopy. Obstet Gynecol Clin North Am. 2004;31:641-54.
18. Orhue AA, Aziken ME, Igbefoh JO. A comparison of two adjunctive treatments for intrauterine adhesions following lysis. Int J Gynaecol Obstet. 2003;82:49-56.
19. Amer MI, El Nadim A, Karim H. The role of intrauterine balloon after hysteroscopy in the prevention of intrauterine adhesions: a prospective controlled study. MEFS J. 2005;10:125-9.
20. Burns JW, Skinner K, Colt J, Sheidlin A, Bronson R, Yaacobi Y, et al. Prevention of tissue injury and postsurgical adhesions by precoating tissue with hyaluronic acid solutions. J Surg Res. 1995;59:644-52.
21. Kim T, Ahn KH, Choi DS, Hwang KJ, Lee BI, Jung MH, et al. A randomized multicentre clinical trial to assess the efficacy and safety of alginate carboxymethylcellulosehyaluronic acid compared to carboxymethylcellulose hyaluronic acid to prevent postoperative intrauterine adhesions. J Minim Invasive Gynecol. 2012;19(6):731-6.
22. Magos A. Hysteroscopic treatment of Asherman syndrome. Reprod Biomed Online. 2002;4 (Suppl 3):46-51.

Chapter 9

Submucous Myoma: Best Possible Ways

Ricardo Bassil Lasmar, Bernardo Portugal Lasmar

■ INTRODUCTION

The first reports of hysteroscopic myomectomy date back to 1978 when Neuwirth successfully removed four uterine fibroids from the uterine cavity. In 1986, Goldrath addressed submucosal fibroids that were entirely intracavitary via the vaginal route, using only grasping forceps.[1] In 2001, Lasmar presented the possibility of removing submucosal fibroids with intramural components hysteroscopically, also acting mechanically on the nodule by enucleating the lesion, separating the fibroid from the pseudocapsule.[2]

Uterine leiomyomas are the most common tumors of the uterus and female pelvis. They are benign nodules primarily composed of smooth muscle cells associated with varying amounts of fibrous connective tissue. According to Muller and Ludovici,[3] they originate from smooth muscle cells, and according to Townsend,[4] they have a unicellular origin. They are well defined but not encapsulated lesions. It is difficult to determine their exact incidence, although it has been cited and accepted as present in 50% of autopsy examinations. They account for approximately one-third of gynecological hospital admissions. They have the highest incidence in nulliparous women and among Black women. Patients often have a family history. Regarding etiology, it can be said that there are conflicting studies suggesting that both estrogen and progesterone may play a role in their development and growth.[5-7] In the early stages of development, they are all intramural, but as they grow, they can remain intramural or extend internally or externally, becoming submucosal or subserosal, respectively. The incidence of leiomyosarcoma is 0.1%, and the sarcomatous degeneration is debatable.[8]

They are more common during the reproductive years when symptoms and dimensions are more significant. In postmenopause, fibroids decrease in size. Most patients are asymptomatic and do not require treatment, only periodic monitoring. In submucosal fibroids, the symptomatology is more pronounced, often leading to surgery. The most common complaint is abnormal uterine bleeding (AUB), in some cases with associated anemia.[9] AUB is often caused by the rupture of dilated vessels on the nodule's surface. In the case of large tumors, an enlarged uterine cavity would create a larger surface area for menstrual shedding. Intramural fibroids would impede venous return, leading to heavy bleeding. Fibroids can also alter the production of local endometrial factors, such as prostaglandins. Falcone[10] theorizes the occurrence of vascular changes in the endometrium and myometrium. Fibroids would cause vascular ectasias through compression mechanisms and the local action of growth factors. There is also dyspareunia, abdominal discomfort, a sensation of heaviness, as well as lower abdominal cramp-like pain, during or outside the menstrual period. They can also be a cause of infertility. When, for some reason, submucosal fibroids undergo degenerative changes, characteristic signs and symptoms of inflammation appear, such as pain, fever, foul-smelling discharge, and abdominal distension.

■ TYPES AND CLASSIFICATION

Fibroids can be located anywhere in the uterus. Depending on their location, they are classified as submucosal (partially or entirely within the uterine cavity), intramural (occupying the myometrium), or subserosal (located partially or entirely on the outer surface of the uterus).

For didactic and practical purposes, the International Federation of Gynecology and Obstetrics (FIGO)[11] has classified fibroids with graphical representation and numerical reference. Starting at 0 for fibroids entirely within the uterine cavity and going up to 7 for those entirely on the external portion of the uterus (**Fig. 1**).

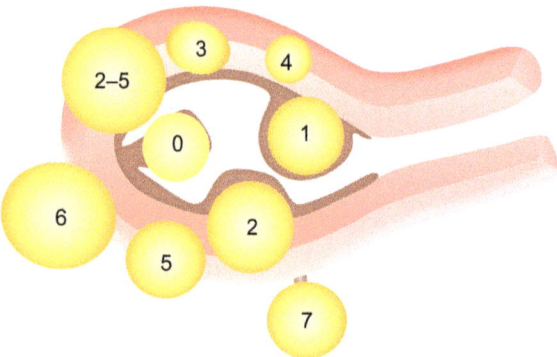

Fig. 1: *International Federation of Gynecology and Obstetrics (FIGO) myoma classification:* Regarding submucosal fibroids (FIGO classification 0 to 4), where hysteroscopic myomectomy is possible, the complexity of the surgery can be assessed using one of two classifications: (1) European Society for Gynaecological Endoscopy classification and (2) Lasmar classification—STEPW.[12]

The classification of submucosal fibroids aims to standardize diagnoses, allowing for the evaluation of therapeutic outcomes and surgical prognosis. The most commonly used classification is that of the European Society for Gynaecological Endoscopy (ESGE), which evaluates the degree of penetration of the submucosal fibroid into the myometrium.[13] The more of the submucosal nodule is located within the myometrium, the higher the grade on the scale, and consequently, the more difficult the surgical treatment. This assessment allows for the consideration of one or more surgical interventions, the need for analog use, the prognosis of the surgery, and the feasibility of hysteroscopic myomectomy. This classification is simple and objective, divided into **(Table 1)**:

- *ESGE classification:* In 2005, Lasmar et al. published a new classification for submucosal fibroids called the "STEPW" classification. This classification is more efficient in assessing the degree of difficulty and the feasibility of hysteroscopic myomectomy. It uses five parameters:
  1. *Size:* Score 0 for nodules up to 2 cm, score 1 for 2–5 cm, and score 2 for >5 cm
  2. *Location (topography):* Score 0 for the lower third of the uterine cavity, score 1 for the middle third, and score 2 for the upper third.
  3. *Extension of the base in relation to the affected wall (extension):* Score 0 for one-third or less of the wall affected, score 1 for one-third to two-thirds of the wall, and score 2 for more than two-thirds of the wall.
  4. *Penetration into the myometrium (penetration):* Score 0—myoma totally inside the uterine cavity, score 1—major part of the myoma inside the cavity, and score 2—major part of myoma inside of the myometrium
  5. *Uterine wall (wall):* Score 0 for anterior and posterior wall fibroids, score 1 for lateral wall fibroids.

All these parameters are recorded in a spreadsheet with their respective scores, which are then summed to determine the final score for the fibroid. The classification is applied to each individual nodule, and the final score indicates the feasibility of technically achievable myomectomy, complex myomectomy, or likely impossibility of the procedure. In schematic terms, it is possible to describe the classification table for submucosal fibroids using the abbreviations STEPW **(Table 2)**.

- *Lasmar classification—STEPW*

TABLE 1: ESGE classification.

Type	Intramural penetration of myoma
0	Totally in uterine cavity
1	>50% in uterine cavity
2	<50% in uterine cavity

(ESGE: European Society for Gynaecological Endoscopy)

TABLE 2: Lasmar classification: STEPW.

Score	Size	Topography	Extension of the base	Penetration	Wall	Total
0	≤2 cm	Lower	≤/3	0	+1	
1	>2 to 5 cm	Middle	>1/3 to 2/3	≤50%		
2	>5 cm	Upper	>2/3	>50%		
Total score	+	+	+	+		=

Score	Group	Suggested treatment
0–4	I	Low complexity hysteroscopic myomectomy
5–6	II	Complex hysteroscopic myomectomy, consider preparing with GnRH
7–9	III	Recommend and alternative nonhysteroscopic technique

(GnRH: gonadotropin-releasing hormone)

DIAGNOSIS AND PLANNING

In the medical history, abnormal uterine bleeding (AUB) during menstruation or outside of it is the most common complaint, as well as dysmenorrhea. Infertility and, especially, recurrent miscarriages may be related to submucosal fibroids. Ultrasonography (US) allows for the identification of the tumor within the uterine cavity, and in some cases, suspicion arises during hysterosalpingography performed during infertility investigations. Transvaginal ultrasonography (TVUS) provides information on the number of nodules, their dimensions, location, the possibility of an intramural component of the submucosal fibroid, and the investigation of uterine adnexa.

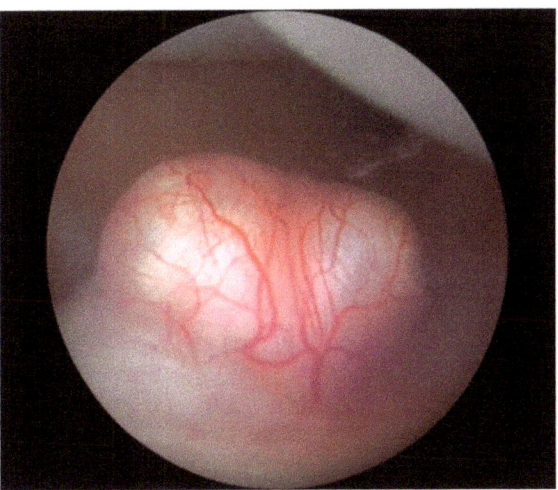

Fig. 2: Vision of submucous myoma in hysteroscopy.

Hysteroscopy (HSC) confirms the diagnosis of intracavitary nodules, providing a detailed description of the fibroid, its size, base dimension, location, number, suspicion of degeneration, and intramural component **(Fig. 2)**. Hysteroscopy can identify associated diseases and, most importantly, the appearance of the endometrium, which often appears hypertrophic. Directed or guided biopsy of the endometrium or associated lesion completes the investigation and confirms the existence of benign uterine disease only. There is no need to biopsy the fibroid nodule, as hysteroscopic visualization is sufficient for diagnosis.

Hysterosonography (HSG) adds important information to the preoperative investigation of submucosal fibroids with an intramural component, revealing the degree of penetration of the fibroid into the myometrium and the measurement of free myometrium between the nodule and the serosa. However, it does not allow for histopathological examination in cases of associated pathologies such as polyps or endometrial hyperplasia.

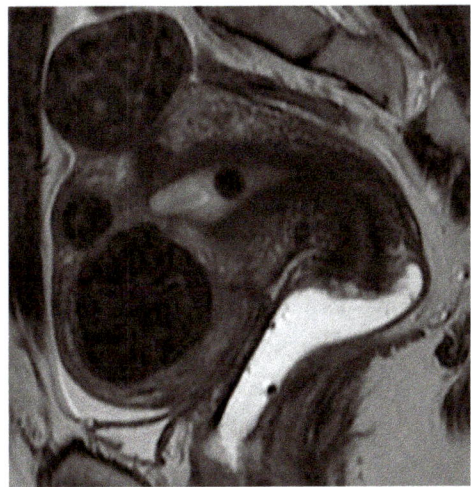

Fig. 3: Magnetic resonance imaging of the uterus with submucous, intramural, and subserosal myoma.

Pelvic magnetic resonance imaging (MRI) can assist in the diagnosis of other causes of AUB, especially adenomyosis **(Fig. 3)**.[14] It can determine all nodules, the degree of fibroid penetration into the myometrium, and the amount of free myometrium to the serosa with greater accuracy. As it is precise in studying uterine walls, it allows for the diagnosis of adenomyosis by evaluating the junctional zone, indicating that AUB may persist even after myomectomy. MRI, by locating smaller fibroids, can anticipate the possibility of the "recurrence" of an extra- or intracavitary lesion. This would demonstrate that this new fibroid already existed at the time of surgery and did not occur after therapy.

Hysteroscopy allows for the differential diagnosis of submucosal fibroids with intramural fibroids compressing the cavity, fibrous endometrial polyps, embryonic remnants, and endometrial adenocarcinoma. The texture, consistency, surface, vascular appearance, and coloration of submucosal fibroids are very characteristic, allowing for a diagnosis even when biopsy is not performed **(Fig. 4)**. During hysteroscopy, submucosal fibroids appear as white, hard tumors with a smooth or bosselated surface, with numerous dilated vessels on the surface.

Intramural fibroids, deforming the uterine cavity, have a more similar appearance to focal endometrial thickening. During hysteroscopy, moving the tip of the hysteroscopic sheath over the endometrium covering the bulge identifies a white and hard nodule. Fibrous sessile polyps have a similar appearance and consistency to submucosal fibroids. The vascular pattern on the lesion's surface, palpation with forceps, and directed biopsy help

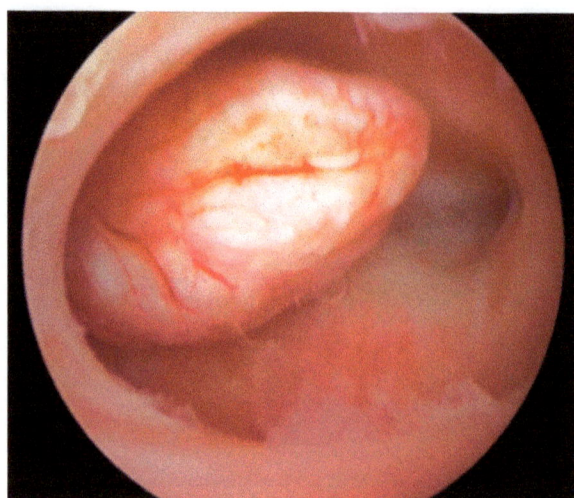

Fig. 4: Submucous myoma in cornual place.

establish the diagnosis. Degenerated submucosal fibroids appear hysteroscopically as a yellowish–white, fibroelastic lesion with softened and irregular areas, sometimes friable, resembling endometrial cancer and infected embryonic remnants. Histopathological examination is essential.

The most challenging differential diagnosis during hysteroscopy is with adenomyoma. Adenomyoma appears white, with a hardened consistency similar to fibroids. Fibroids coexist with adenomyosis in about 30% of cases, usually diffuse adenomyosis, contributing to the globular appearance of the uterus.

OPERATIVE TIPS

Several observations are important for the performance of hysteroscopic myomectomy:

- Always perform ambulatory hysteroscopy before surgery and compare it with imaging examinations. This way, each submucosal fibroid can be classified, allowing for appropriate and accurate surgical planning.
- In patients with infertility, after complete fibroid removal, ambulatory hysteroscopy should be performed in two to three menstrual cycles after surgery.
- Clinically and hemodynamically stabilize the patient before surgery.
- Place a Foley catheter in bladder, in all hospital-based myomectomies to monitor fluid balance and identify early bladder perforation.
- Familiarize yourself with and identify complications, especially bleeding, uterine perforation, and overload.
- During surgery, maintain constant visibility of the cavity and only use energy when the location is visually identified. If visibility of the cavity is lost and cannot be recovered, evaluate and investigate the possibility of perforation. In cases of using electrical current, it is imperative to investigate the pelvic and abdominal cavities.

The location of the fibroid may increase the complexity of hysteroscopic myomectomy. For example:

- Cervical fibroids can obstruct distension and visibility. In such cases, focusing on the base of the lesion and enucleating it may be the best option. However, for large volumes, slicing to reduce volume could facilitate enucleation.
- Fibroids located in the lateral uterine wall, especially those with an intramural component, increase the risks due to proximity to major vessels. Attention to hemostasis and fluid balance is essential. The possibility of a two-stage surgery should always be evaluated.
- Fibroids in the fundal region impede the movement of the resectoscope and nodule mobilization. Different approaches should be attempted, using the Collins loop in various positions, which can facilitate enucleation.
- Cornual fibroids present the same difficulties as fundal fibroids, with the added complication of having an additional adjacent wall blocking surgical instrument movement. This thinner wall increases the risk of perforation and intestinal loop injury with an intact uterus due to heat dissipation.

WHICH INSTRUMENT AND WHEN

Office Myomectomy

In office hysteroscopy, scissors should be used for direct access to the fibroid's base, creating small incisions around the fibroid until the pseudocapsule is reached. Subsequently, with lateral and inferior movements, progressive release of the lesion is performed, cutting only through fibrous trabeculae found. With this enucleation technique, bleeding is minimal or absent since it does not interfere with the vascularization of the myometrium or the fibroid's surface.

The limit for ambulatory myomectomy is the patient's pain threshold and fibroids Group I of Lasmar classification.[15]

It is important to highlight that the procedure can be interrupted at any time without risk to the patient. The removal of the fibroid from the uterine cavity after enucleation of the uterine wall is possible in cases where the nodule's diameter is smaller than the internal orifice. Larger fibroids may remain in the uterine cavity and are often eliminated spontaneously until the next menstrual period. The presence of a free-floating fibroid in the uterine cavity does not pose any risk to the patient and only requires a follow-up hysteroscopy after menstruation for evaluation.

Hospital Myomectomy

In hospital myomectomy, for fibroids of Lasmar's Group I that were not suitable for ambulatory treatment and Group II, anesthesia is used, with sedation for Group I and a block for Group II.

The technique is similar, using a mono- or bipolar resectoscope, cutting current, and the Collins loop **(Fig. 5)**. An incision is made around the fibroid, seeking the pseudocapsule. Subsequently, with lateral movements between the fibroid and pseudocapsule, the nodule is progressively released until complete enucleation. Afterward, the fibroid is longitudinally resected using the same Collins loop, followed by slicing with the semicircular loop for its removal from the uterine cavity.[16]

In summary, with the Collins loop, an incision is made around the fibroid, the pseudocapsule is found, enucleation is performed, and slicing begins. The fibroid is removed from the uterine wall. Hemostasis can be achieved with a coagulation current if needed.

■ UPDATES

Tissue removal devices have been increasingly gaining prominence in the approach to submucosal fibroids. They utilize a rotary blade for resection and suction tubing to remove tissue fragments. With the evolution of the instruments, which have become smaller in diameter and equipped with reusable (permanent) blades, it has become a cost-effective option with the possibility of use in an outpatient setting.

Ultrasound-guided radiofrequency ablation (RFA) of fibroids is a technique that can be accomplished using a hysteroscopic or, more commonly, laparoscopic approach.

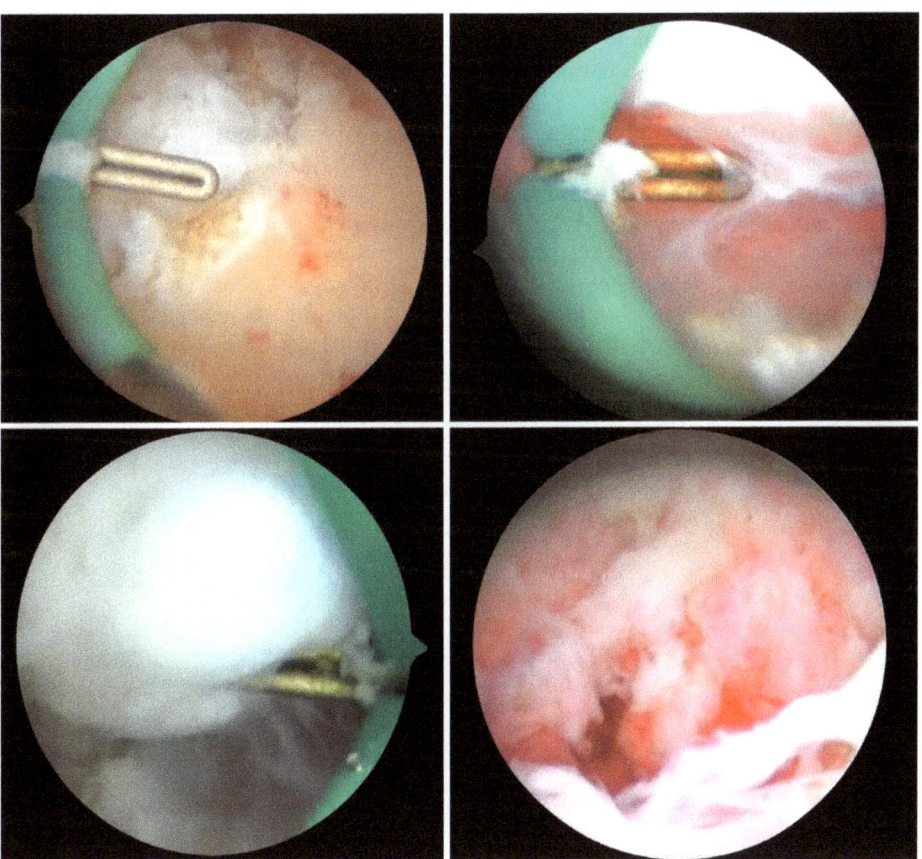

Fig. 5: Myoma enucleation using Collins loop.

Transcervical resection, using the operating channel of the hysteroscope, allows for the approach to fibroids with large intramural components or even adenomyosis. Ultrasonographic control is important whenever there is intervention in the deep myometrium.

CONCLUSION

The complexity of hysteroscopic myomectomy is due to several factors. Therefore, classifying the fibroid before surgery and understanding the patient's desire for pregnancy are crucial for the procedure's success. In Group II fibroids according to Lasmar, it is possible to encounter cases where multiple surgeries are required for complete fibroid removal, with lower risk.

The surgical technique of directly approaching the fibroid's base, both in outpatient and inpatient settings, and leaving the nodule to be expelled later or sliced without vascularization, in the hospital, reduces the operative time, bleeding, and the risk of overload, making the surgery safe.

REFERENCES

1. Neuwirth RS. A new technique and additional experience with hysteroscopic resection of submucous fibroids. Am J Obstet Gynecol. 1978;131:91-4.
2. Lasmar RB, Barrozo PM. Histeroscopia uma abordagem prática. Editora Médsi, 2001.
3. Miller NF, Ludovici PP. On the origin and development of uterine fibroids. Am J Obstet Gynecol. 1955;70(4):720-40.
4. Townsend DE, Sparkes RS, Baluda MC, McClelland G. Unicellular histogenesis of uterine leiomyomas as determined by electrophoresis by glucose-6-phosphate dehydrogenase. Am J Obstet Gynecol. 1970;107(8):1168-73.
5. Tinelli A, Vinciguerra M, Malvasi A, Andjić M, Babović I, Sparić R. Uterine Fibroids and Diet. Int J Environ Res Public Health. 2021;18(3):1066.
6. Sparic R, Mirkovic L, Malvasi A, Tinelli A. Epidemiology of Uterine Myomas: A Review. Int J Fertil Steril. 2016;9(4):424-35.
7. Cheng MH, Wang PH. Uterine myoma: a condition amenable to medical therapy? Expert Opin Emerg Drugs. 2008;13(1):119-33.
8. Devaud N, Vornicova O, Abdul Razak AR, Khalili K, Demicco EG, Mitric C, et al. Leiomyosarcoma: Current Clinical Management and Future Horizons. Surg Oncol Clin N Am. 2022;31(3):527-46.
9. Puri K, Famuyide AO, Erwin PJ, Stewart EA, Laughlin-Tommaso SK. Submucosal fibroids and the relation to heavy menstrual bleeding and anemia. Am J Obstet Gynecol. 2014;210:38.e1.
10. Falcone T, Gustilo AM. Minimally invasive surgery for mass lesions. Clin Obstet Gynecol. 2005;48(2):353-60.
11. Kahveci B, Budak MS, Ege S, Obut M, Bağlı I, Oğlak SC, et al. PALM-COEIN classification system of FIGO VS the classic terminology in patients with abnormal uterine bleeding. Ginekol Pol. 2021;92(4):257-61.
12. Lasmar RB, Barrozo PR, Dias R, Oliveira MA. Submucous myomas: a new presurgical classification to evaluate the viability of hysteroscopic surgical treatment--preliminary report. J Minim Invasive Gynecol. 2005;12(4):308-11.
13. Wamsteker K, Emanuel MH, deKruif JH. Transcervical hysteroscopic resection of submucous fibroids for abnormal uterine bleeding: Results regarding degree of intramural extension. Obstet Gynecol. 1993;82:736-40.
14. Vilos GA, Allaire C, Laberge PY, Leyland N, Vilos AG, Murji A, et al. The management of uterine leiomyomas. J Obstet Gynaecol Can. 2015;37(2):157-81.
15. Lasmar RB, Lasmar BP. Limiting factors of office hysteroscopic myomectomy. In: Tinelli A, Alonso Pacheco L, Haimovich S (Eds). Hysteroscopy. Cham: Springer; 2018.
16. Lasmar RB, Barrozo PRM, da Rosa DB, Lasmar BP, Modotte WP, Dias R. Hysteroscopic myomectomy in a submucous fibroid near from tubal ostia and 5 mm from the serosa: a case report from the Endoscopy Service of Ginendo-RJ. Gynecol Surg. 2009;6:283-6.

Chronic Endometritis, Tuberculosis, and Hysteroscopy

Chapter 10

Sushma Deshmukh

Tuberculosis and chronic endometritis
– A hidden enemy
Affects reproduction badly
Silent killer & intruder!
It can be an accidental detection
We have to use clinical acumen
Unexplained infertility, RIF, RPL
Sometimes no symptoms/no complain
Something wrong, something odd
Leaving us confused
As someone somewhere,
A master player –
Affecting gestosis.
Think tuberculosis/chronic endometritis

CHRONIC ENDOMETRITIS

Introduction

It is an asymptomatic condition. Endometritis is an inflammation of the endometrial mucosa. In the last years, a growing scientific interest has been focused on chronic endometritis (CE) and on the consequences of this pathology on reproduction. Incidence is 0.2–46% among infertile women.

But one of the major problems in diagnosing CE is that the medical fraternity is not enough aware of this entity.

Etiology

Chlamydia trachomatis (Chlamydia), *Neisseria gonorrhoeae* (gonorrhea), group B *Streptococcus*, *Mycoplasma hominis*, tuberculosis, and various viruses are causes of endometritis unrelated to pregnancy. Sometimes immunological factors are also there.

Why we are worried?
- In patients of recurrent implantation failure, CE was identified in 30.3% with low implantation rate of 11.5%.
- Due its ceiled nature, a great variability ranging from 30 to 60% of patients with repeated implantation failure in assisted reproductive technique (ART)
- About 50–60% of women with recurrent pregnancy losses (RPL)

Diagnosis of CE is challenging. Why?
- Clinically, the presence of CE is frequently overlooked as this pathology is poorly known by many specialists and because it lacks specific symptoms.
- In fact, in many cases, CE is asymptomatic or it may cause abnormal uterine bleeding, pain, infertility, and ART failures.
- Many times it is diagnosed accidently during hysteroscopy.

Evaluation, Diagnosis, and Management

- Laboratory tests—for chlamydia nowadays polymerase chain reaction (PCR) giving good results.
- Histology is considered the gold standard for diagnosing CE based on plasma cell detection but it remains an operator-dependent technique.

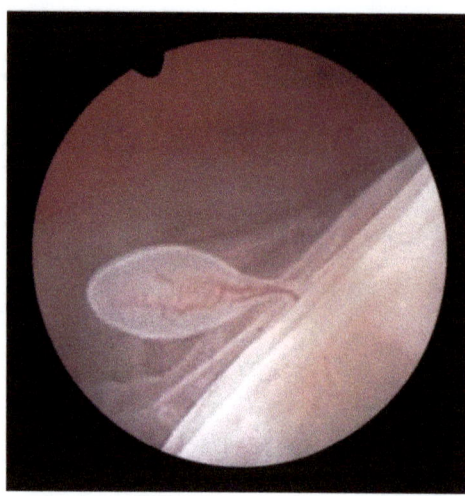

Fig. 1: Hysteroscopic picture of micropolyp.

- Recently, CD138 immunohistochemistry staining for plasma cells has provided higher diagnostic accuracy, sensitivity as compared to hematoxylin and eosin (H&E) analysis. However, even after interpretation of CD138 immunohistochemistry staining, no consensus exists, because tuberculosis GeneXpert is more sensitive test.
- *Ultrasonography:* 3D ultrasound was performed revealing the presence of several isoechogenic round well limited structures inside the endometrial cavity[1] but not confirmatory.
- *Hysteroscopy:* It is a reliable technique for diagnosing CE. Main hysteroscopic features are given below:[2]
    - *Micropolyps*: These are pedunculated translucent structures <1 mm in size, sporadic isolated structures or occur in clusters, anywhere in the cavity **(Fig. 1)**
    - Focal hyperemia
    - The endometrium may appear whitish and irregularly thick due to increased stromal edema
    - *Undulating or pseudopolypoid endometrium:* The undulating nature of the endometrium is best appreciated with the hysteroscope making an angle of about 45° with the endometrium.
    - *Strawberry appearance and hyperemia:* The endometrial gland openings appear intense whitish and surrounded by intense hyperemia thereby giving a strawberry-like appearance
    - Endometrial hemorrhagic spots
    - Tuberculosis of the endometrial cavity.

Management: Doxycycline 100 mg orally for 21 days with tablet metrogyl 400 mg twice a day for 5 days or clindamycin 300 mg.

TUBERCULOSIS AND HYSTEROSCOPY

Introduction

Tuberculosis (TB) has been a major cause of illness and death worldwide for ages and still continues to be so as a major health problem. Genital tuberculosis (GTB) causes significant pelvic morbidity due to uterine adhesions and infertility in developing countries. Hysteroscopy is a useful modality in diagnosing endometrial TB. It plays an important role in evaluation of uterine cavity and is of immense help in infertility as well as in reproductive failure.

Genital tuberculosis is a disease of no symptoms or masquerades as other gynecological conditions. Most of the times, it is discovered while investigating infertile patient. Among all countries, two-thirds of the cases are in India (27%).[3]

Incidence

It is estimated that 5–13% of all pulmonary TB patients develop genital involvement. Genital TB is responsible for 5% of all pelvic infections. This infection has been implicated in 5–10% of infertility cases.

Genital organs most frequently affected by tuberculosis in order of frequency are fallopian tubes (95–100%), endometrium (50–60%), ovaries (20–30%), cervix (5–15%), and rarely vulva and vagina (1–2%).[4]

Given the hormone-dependent nature of the female genital tuberculosis, 90% of cases involve women under 40 years of age.

Endometrial Tuberculosis

Grossly the size and shape of the uterus may appear normal. The tuberculous process generally is localized to the endometrium, is most extensive in the fundus, and decreases toward the cervix. The myometrium is not usually involved.

Clinical Presentation

Majority of patients are in the reproductive group. 75% being in 20–45 year age group. Postmenopausal women amount for 7–11% of genital tuberculosis.[5] Clinical presentations are infertility, amenorrhea, increased miscarriage rates, and chronic pelvic pain.

Diagnosis

Being a paucibacillary disease, demonstration of *Mycobacterium tuberculosis* is not possible in all cases.

Various blood tests, nonspecific tests, serological, and sonoradiological investigations such as USG, HSG, and MRI tried to diagnose this disease. Nowadays, CBNAAT-GeneXpert with Culture (Sample collected in normal saline) and histopathological study (in Formalin) done from collected from endometrium giving good predictive value.

Hysteroscopy

Hysteroscopy is a useful modality in diagnosing endometrial TB. The best time for conducting hysteroscopic examination is in premenstrual phase so that any overlying deposits are not missed out.

There can be difficulties since beginning, i.e., from the entry of hysteroscope through the external orifice till the negotiation through cervical canal, internal os to the uterine cavity.

Most of the times, entry is easy. With the help of 2.9-mm hysteroscope, we can enter through the external orifice with little difficulty.

Difficulties at External Cervical Orifice

We need to negotiate through the external cervical orifice with the help of 2.9-mm hysteroscope and semirigid 5-Fr seizures and forceps. We can resect the fibrous tissue **(Fig. 2)** or ring and advance further under hysteroscopic guidance.

Difficulties at Cervical Canal

Mild flimsy adhesions can be dissected and cut by blunt adhesiolysis with 2.9-mm hysteroscope with 5-Fr scissors. We can get varied pictures of adhesions. With proper visualization and persistent controlled pressure, distension we can proceed with the help of scissors and forceps under vision. We can also use bipolar current to dissect tough adhesions.

- Sometimes, we may not get the typical picture of the cervical canal of arbor vitae and may get typical blunt cervical canal **(Fig. 3)**
- Sometimes filmy adhesions with tubercles **(Fig. 4)**
- Thickened fibrous tissue **(Fig. 5)**

Difficulties at Internal Cervical Orifice

The internal orifice has an oval shape with a transverse diameter of 4–5 mm in nulliparous and 7–8 mm in multiparous women. We can negotiate easily with 2.9-mm Bettocchi hysteroscope with anterior posterior oval diameter. So we can just rotate the scope and negotiate.

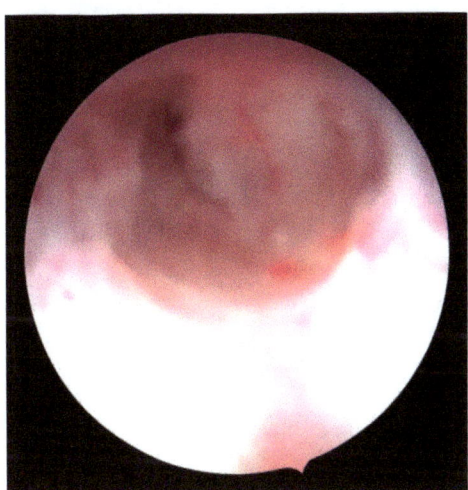

Fig. 3: Blunt cervical canal.

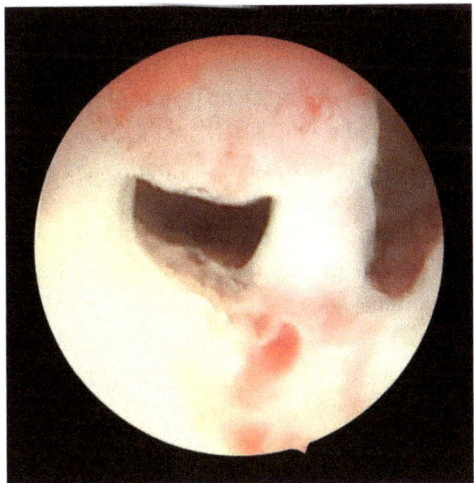

Fig. 2: Fibrous tissue at external cervical os.

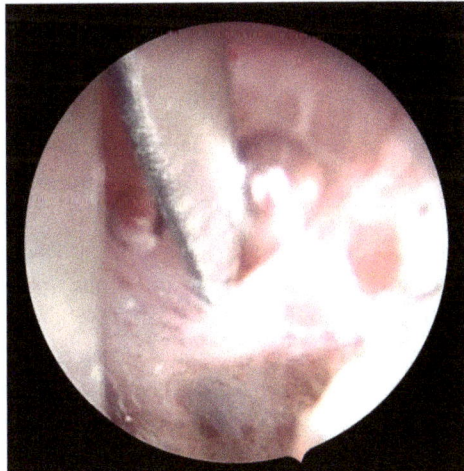

Fig. 4: Filmy adhesions with tubercles.

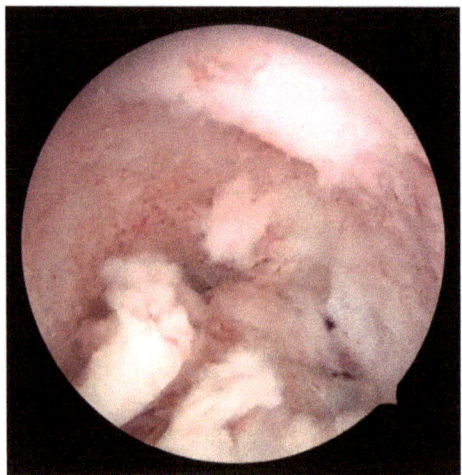

Fig. 5: Thickened fibrous tissue.

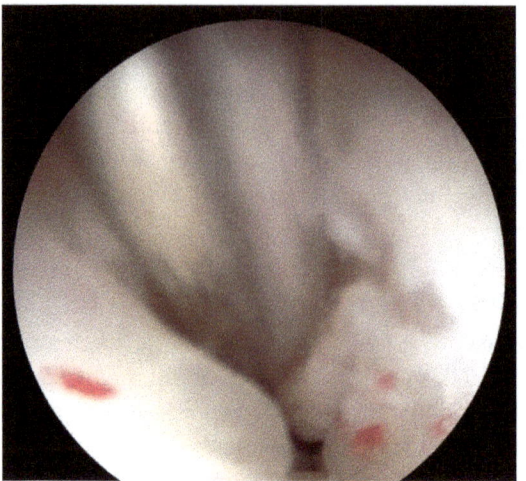

Fig. 7: Breaking and cutting the adhesions.

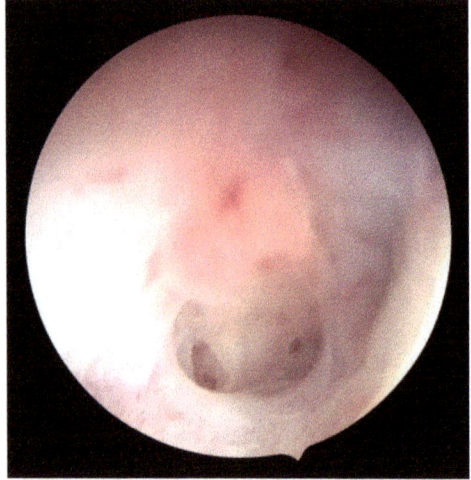

Fig. 6: Fibrosis at internal orifice.

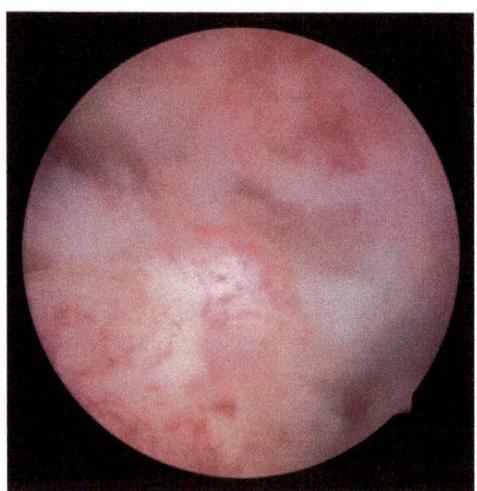

Fig. 8: Bizarre dirty endometrium.

In GTB, there can be adhesions and fibrosis (**Fig. 6**) at internal orifice. With the help of scissors, we can break and cut the adhesions (**Fig. 7**).

In the cavity: In 70% infertile patients with GTB, cavity is normal with bilateral open ostia and normal looking endometrium. Classical hysteroscopic findings of endometrial TB is a rough dirty looking bizarre pale endometrium (**Fig. 8**) with gland openings not seen and with overlying whitish deposits.

However, all these signs may not be seen in the same case. Various presentations can be seen. One should be well versed with it.

The findings can be:
- Rough endometrial surface in late proliferative phase
- The endometrium may be pale looking (**Fig. 9**), thin, irregular with or without focal areas of hyperemia.
- It may be partially or almost completely covered by multiple irregular whitish deposits.
- Whitish deposits are the most pathognomonic of TB; however, they may not be always seen.
- These tubercles are often seen on the endometrial surface in the premenstrual phase and are usually located adjacent to the tubal ostia.
- The whitish deposits along with intervening hyperemic endometrium gives a geographical map like appearance (**Fig. 10**).
- Sometimes whitish deposits do not overly the endometrium and instead they are anchored to flimsy adhesions by being impregnated on the same (**Fig. 11**).

Chronic Endometritis, Tuberculosis, and Hysteroscopy

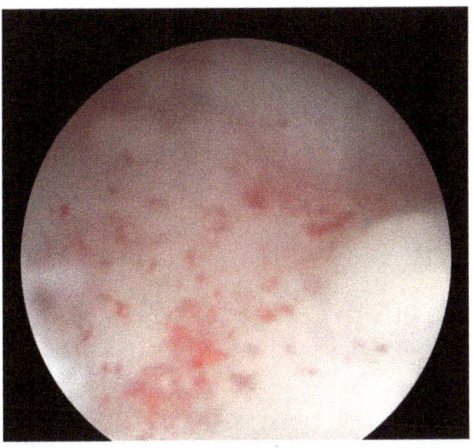

Fig. 9: Irregular pale endometrium with hyperemia at places.

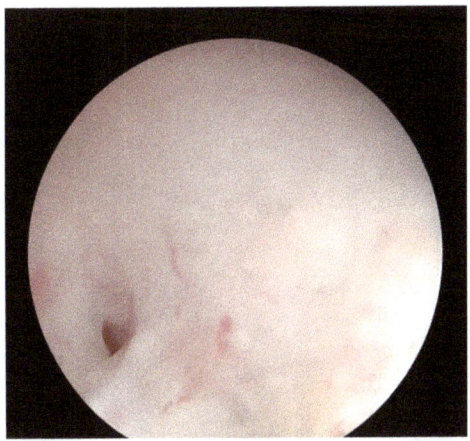

Fig. 12: Right ostium adhesions with pale endometrium.

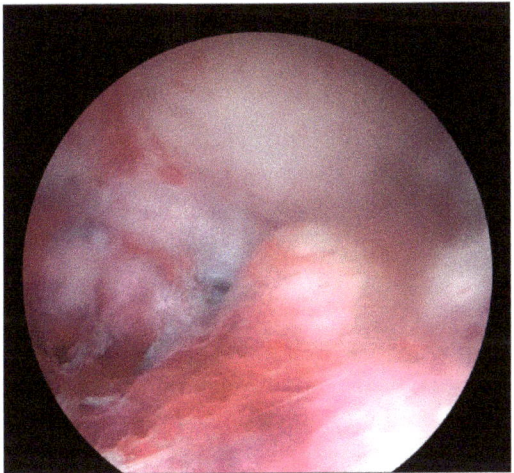

Fig. 10: The whitish deposits along with intervening hyperemic endometrium.

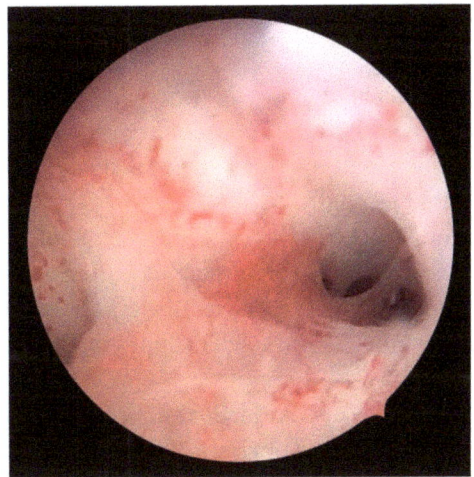

Fig. 13: Left ostium covered with flimsy adhesions.

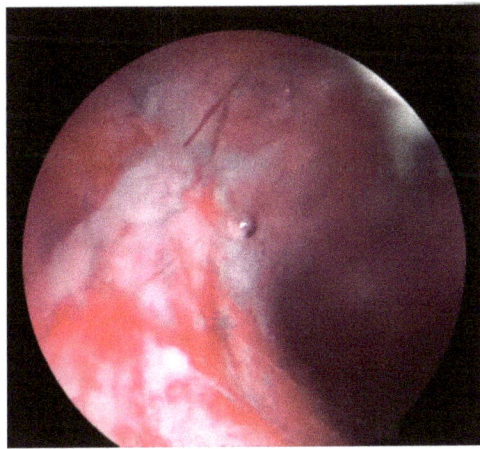

Fig. 11: Rough dirty looking endometrium—flimsy adhesions with tubercle.

These flimsy adhesions are not shed in menstruation hence the impregnated deposits are seen even in postmenstrual phase.
- Sometimes tubal ostial fibrosis (**Fig. 12**) and adhesions are seen so tubal ostia may be blocked or may not be visible on hysteroscopy. We can appreciate intraluminal adhesions in the interstitial part of the tube by placing the microhysteroscope tip very close to tubal orifice and viewing with a source magnification (**Fig. 13**).
- Endocervical scarring is also seen in endometrial TB
- Granulomas may be present rarely.
- Synechiae when present in the absence of intervention—pale looking cavity partially or completely obliterated by adhesions of varying degree

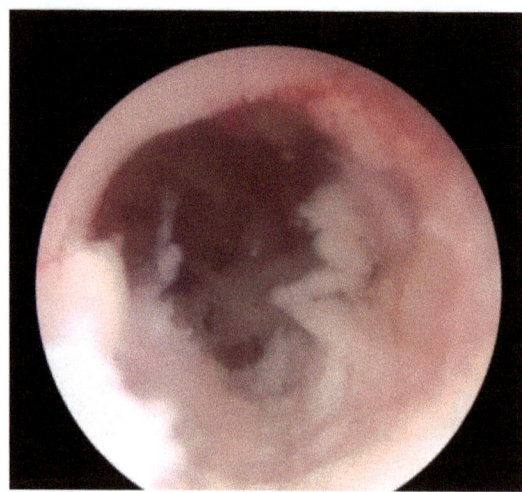

Fig. 14: View of uterine cavity from internal orifice—shrunken small cavity.

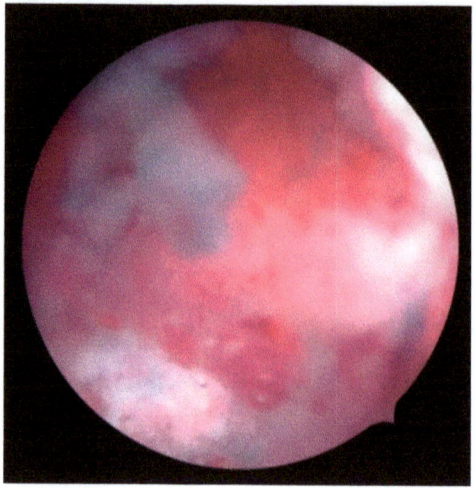

Fig. 15: After instillation of methylene blue and the white deposits.

- Poor distensibility
- Caseation and ulceration occur in the advanced stage which may lead to adhesion or synechiae formation (Asherman's syndrome)
- The whitish deposits vary in size, have irregular borders, and peel off easily when touched with hysteroscope. Even in the advanced pelvic tuberculosis, evidence of caseation fibrosis and calcification is rarely seen in the uterine cavity.
- The cavity may appear small and shrunken (**Fig. 14**).
- Very occasionally the cavity is obliterated by extensive fibrosis.
- *Starry sky appearance:* Sometimes whitish deposits are not seen. But with vital staining with methylene blue (chromopertubation), such deposits are seen, thereby giving starry sky appearance[6] (**Fig. 15**). Most of the time, we get various types of presentations depending upon the severity.

Role of Therapeutic and Second Look Hysteroscopy

A second look hysteroscopy is necessary to visualize the residual disease in infertile patient. Especially when we are planning for IVF then we can have idea about the status of the endometrium. In such patients, we can do adhesiolysis. Total corporal synechiae due to tuberculosis carries a very poor prognosis following hysteroscopic synechialysis.[7]

Word of Caution

- One has to be careful while performing hysteroscopy in genital TB as cervix is often constricted and negotiation and dilatation with hysteroscope will be difficult.
- There are chances of false passage and perforation.

Advantage of Hysteroscopy

- Visual diagnosis. It is always better to have a look over the endometrium as many times there are false negative histopathological and PCR reports.
- We get an opportunity to get material for histopathological sampling and confirmation of the diagnosis.
- In the same sitting, we can give diagnostic as well as therapeutic benefit to the patient, e.g., adhesiolysis.
- In second look hysteroscopy, we can confirm the benefit of the treatment as well as fertility potential.

CONCLUSION

Genital tuberculosis is a disease of no symptoms. Most of the times, it is discovered during the investigative procedures of infertility.

Hysteroscopy is wonderful modality for diagnostic as well as therapeutic purpose.

REFERENCES

1. Alonso L, Carugno J. Chronic Endometritis: Three-dimensional Ultrasound and Hysteroscopy Correlation. J Minim Invasive Gynecol. 2020;27(5):993-4.

2. Cicinelli E, Vitagliano A, Kumar A, Lasmar RB, Bettocchi S, Haimovich S, et al. Unified diagnostic criteria for chronic endometritis at fluid hysteroscopy: proposal and reliability evaluation through an international randomized-controlled observer study. Fertil Steril. 2019;112(1):162-73.e2.
3. Varma T. (2008). Tuberculosis of the Female Genital Tract. [online] Available from: https://www.glowm.com/section-view/heading/Tuberculosis%20of%20the%20Female%20Genital%20Tract/item/34. [Last accessed November, 2023].
4. World Health Organization. (2016). Global Tuberculosis Report 2016. [online] Available from: https://www.who.int/publications/i/item/9789241565394. [Last accessed November, 2023].
5. Jahromi BN, Rarsanezhad ME, Ghane-Shirazi R. Female genital tuberculosis and infertility. Int J Obstet Gynecol. 2001;75:269-72.
6. Kumar A, Kumar A. Hysteroscopic findings of starry sky appearance and impregnated cobwebs in the endometrial tubercolosis. Int J Gynecol Obstet. 2014;126:280-1.
7. Bukulmez O, Yarali H, Gurgan T. Total corporal synechiae due to tuberculosis carry a very poor prognosis following hysteroscopic synechialysis. Hum Reprod. 1999;14(8):1960-1.

Chapter 11: Isthmocele: Smart Use of Hysteroscopy

Mario Franchini, Paolo Casadio, Giampietro Gubbini

■ INTRODUCTION

Isthmocele is defined as an iatrogenic pouch-like defect of the anterior uterine wall at the site of a previous cesarean scar (CS). It is also called cesarean scar defect (CSD), pouch, or niche and, its presence is usually asymptomatic.[1]

■ TYPES AND ETIOLOGY

Depending on the stage of labor, isthmocele can be detected at cervical uterine junction in women who have an elective CS or at medium third and lower part of cervical canal when the cervix has become part of uterine wall in active labor **(Fig. 1)**.

According to Bij de Vaate isthmocele, it has been classified as: triangle, semicircle, rectangle, circle, droplet, and inclusion cysts **(Figs. 2A to F)**.[2]

A number of studies have attempted to identify and categorize factors associated with isthmocele development. Several hypotheses may explain CSD development: impaired wound healing, adhesion formation, inadequate suturing or incomplete closure of the uterine scar due to myometrial closure technique. The last hypothesis that could increase the risk of incomplete healing of the CS incision relates to patient factors such as an increased maternal body mass index, gestational diabetes, and preeclampsia, but all of these require further investigation before firm conclusions can be made.[3]

■ DIAGNOSIS AND PLANNING

Isthmocele appears as a cystic or hypoechoic distortion in the scar when using 2D or 3D transvaginal ultrasound

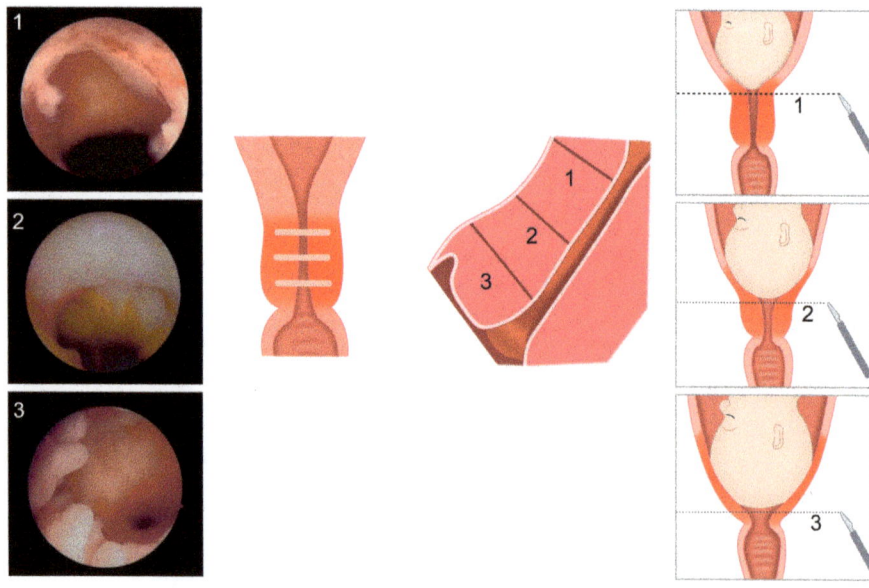

Fig. 1: Isthmocele site can be detected at cervical uterine junction in women who have an elective CS (1), at medium third (2), and lower part of cervical canal (3) when the cervix has become part of uterine wall in active labor. Schematic diagram on the right and hysteroscopic view on the left. (CS: cesarean scar)

(TVUS) with or without saline or gel contrast. Fluid is more likely to be present if the ultrasound is performed between day 7–14 of the cycle, obviating the need for contrast techniques.

Isthmocele is defined as an indentation at the site of the cesarean scar with a depth of at least 2 mm. According to the 2016 practical guideline proposed by European Niche taskforce, basic measurements of isthmocele [length, residual myometrial thickness (RMT), adjacent myometrial thickness (AMT) and depth] should be measured in the sagittal plane. The transverse plane should be considered for the measurement of the width and to identify branches **(Figs. 3A and B)**. On branch basis, CSD can be subclassified as: (1) simple, (2) simple with one branch, (3) complex with more than one branch.

No universal grading standard for the severity of isthmoceles has been established. One way to classify the defect is based on the size of its surface, with grade 1, 2, and 3 corresponding to a surface area of 15 mm^2, 16–25 mm^2, and >25 mm^2, respectively. Other approaches are based on the ratio between the RMT and the AMT. Lastly, a more detailed and complete system includes several factors such as the RMT, the PRM (remaining myometrial thickness/AMT), the number of CS scars, the CS number, and the menstrual conditions that should simultaneously assess.[4]

Isthmocele can be perfectly seen at the time of hysteroscopy under direct vision **(Figs. 4A to F)**. It has been described as a concavity, pouch, sacculation, or wedge at the anterior cervical uterine junction (isthmus) or at the medium lower part of cervical canal. More

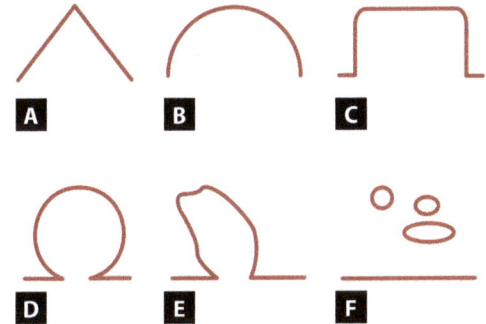

Figs. 2A to F: Schematic diagram to assess isthmocele shape. According to Bij de Vaate iclassification: (A) Triangle; (B) semicircle; (C) rectangle; (D) circle; (E) droplet; (F) inclusion cyst.

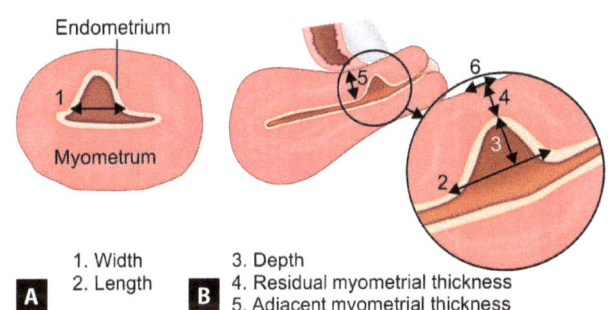

Figs. 3A and B: Basic measurements of isthmocele with transvaginal ultrasound proposed by European Niche Taskforce. (A) Transversal plane; (B) Sagittal view.

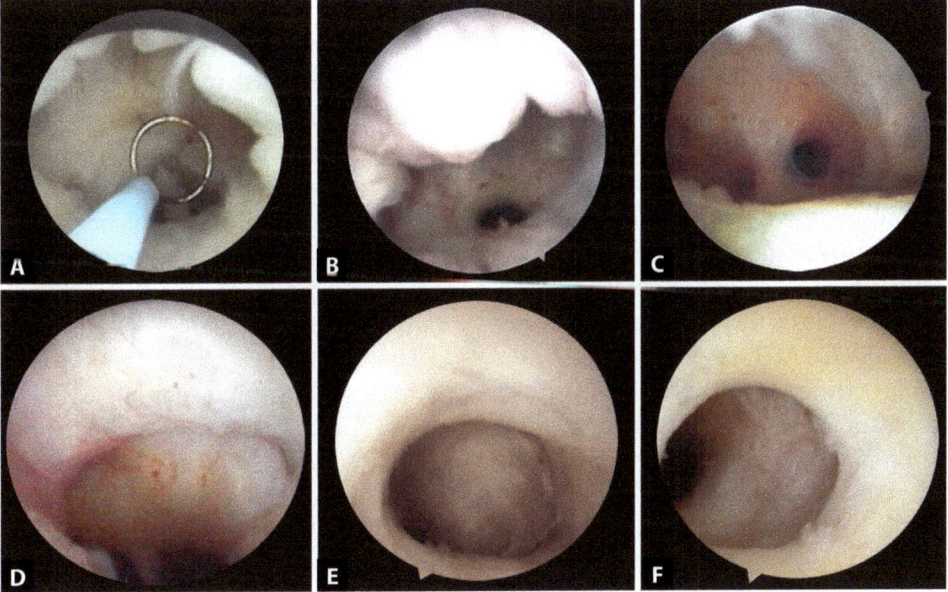

Figs. 4A to F: Isthmocele hysteroscopic appearance.

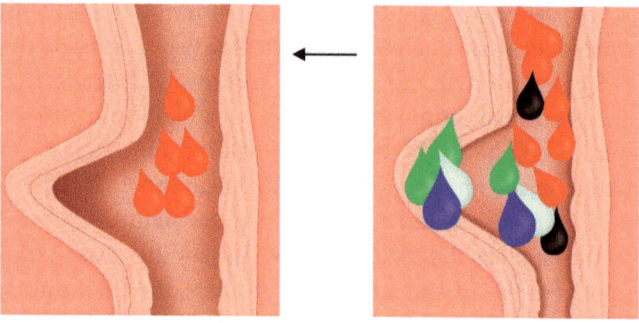

Fig. 5: Flattening effect of hysteroscopic treatment: resection restores the continuity of the cervical canal and improves menstrual drainage reducing blood accumulation in the isthmocele and reflux into the uterine cavity.

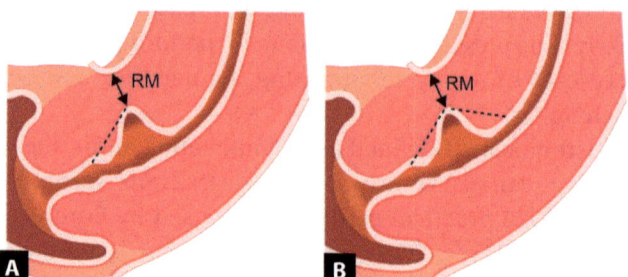

Figs. 6A and B: Hysteroscopic isthmoplasty is performed by resecting only (A) the inferior/proximal rim of the niche (Fabres 2005) or (B) removing the fibrotic tissue of the inferior/proximal and superior/distal of the defect (Gubbini 2008). (RM: residual myometrium)

precisely, isthmocele is usually surrounded by a fibrotic ring, and filled with brown-colored blood and dense viscous mucus-like material during and immediately after menstrual cycle. A careful washing and drainage permit visualization of the surface that appears covered with congested endometrium, capillary dilatation, and inflamed tissue placed in the niche and all around it.

Since isthmocele can lead to abnormal uterine bleeding, dyspareunia, pelvic pain, and infertility, the treatment is predominantly performed to relieve symptoms and to improve fertility. CSD without symptoms or infertility should not be treated.

■ OPERATIVE TIPS

The most common and less invasive treatment to remove excess scar tissue is hysteroscopic approach. The resection, flattening the CSD area, restores the continuity of the cervical canal and improves menstrual drainage reducing blood accumulation in the niche and reflux into the uterine cavity **(Fig. 5)**.

Hysteroscopic channel-like treatment is usually performed with small variations among surgeons, using a 26 or 27 Fr resectoscope. The procedure begins by resecting, with monopolar or bipolar loop, the fibrotic tissue of the inferior/proximal rim of the niche (closest to the external cervical os) **(Fig. 6A)** proposed by Fabres[5] or with superior/distal edge of the defect (closest to the uterine cavity) **(Fig. 6B)** proposed by Gubbini[6] and usually ends, using a roller ball or loop electrode, with coagulation of fragile vessels of the niche ceiling or with superficial coagulation of the entire isthmocele surface.[7]

In recent years, the hysteroscopic procedure has been performed using a 15–16 Fr resectoscope.[8] The first small diameter resectoscope (SDR) was available in 2008. SDR

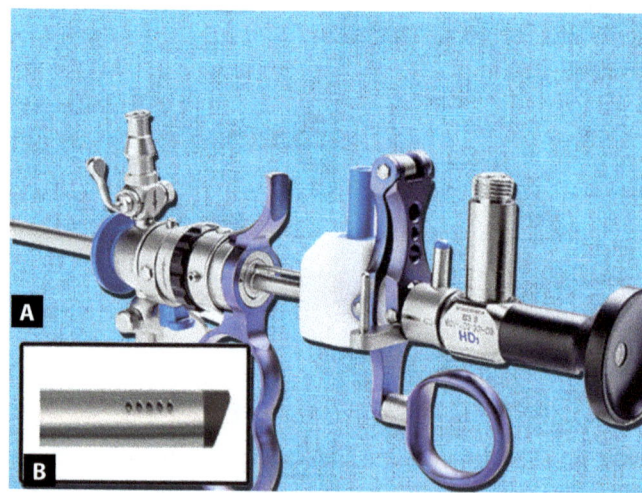

Figs. 7A and B: (A) Mini-hysteroresectoscope 16 Fr (GUBBINI system; Tontarra, Medizintechnik, Tuttlingen, Germany); (B) Oval tip.

systems include the use of 5-Fr bipolar or monopolar HF electrodes and mechanical forceps in a working sheath with 5-Fr operative channel using the same outer sheath with normal saline or nonionic distention media. Leaving the outer sheath inside the cervical canal, the system of sheath connections enables an easy assembly and a smooth exchange during the procedures shifting from 5-Fr instrumentation to miniaturized loop surgery **(Figs. 7 and 8)**.

The SDR allows the surgeon to perform standard maneuvers of resectoscopic CSD treatment with the advantages of miniaturized instrumentation without the complications related to cervical dilation. Therefore, the procedure is performed in the real anatomy of the cervical canal with vaginoscopic approach.

The procedure is generally performed in the operating room, under general anesthesia, with the

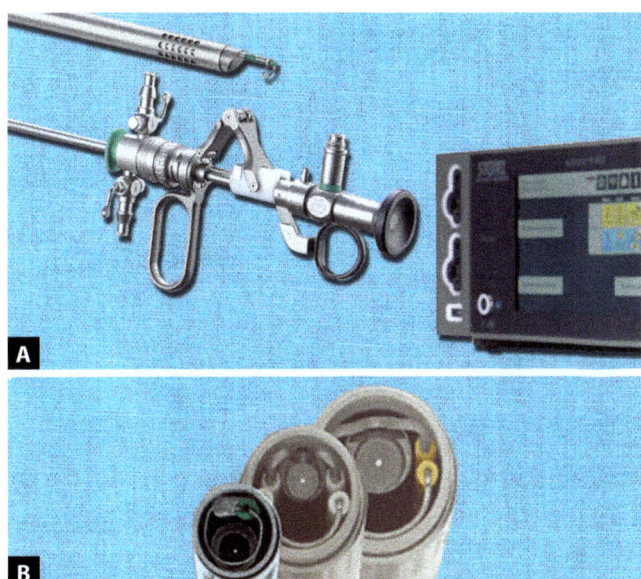

Figs. 8A and B: (A) Mini-resectoscope 15 Fr (Karl Storz SE & Co. KG, Tuttlingen, Germany); (B) Focus on tip sizes 15–22–27 Fr.

patient in the dorsal lithotomy position, during the proliferative phase or under medical pretreatment. The table must be flat; Trendelenburg positioning, that should generally be avoided, could be used during the procedure in acutely anteverted anteflexed canal. As with any gynecologic procedure, the bimanual examination should always be performed before starting to identify any anatomical modifications. An indwelling Foley catheter is not necessary; however, the bladder may be filled with methylene blue solution before starting the procedure.

With the vaginoscopic entry technique, using 15/16-Fr resectoscope, the need for the traditional instruments used for entry with 26/27-Fr resectoscope is avoided. The procedure begins by introducing the hysteroscope into the vagina. The vagina is then distended, and the cervix and external os are usually easily identified. Once the external os is located, the resectoscope is carefully inserted and the isthmocele is localized and visualized after a careful washing and drainage. Finally, the entire uterine cavity should always be inspected.

The procedure begins with the resection of the fibrotic tissue of the proximal (step 1) **(Fig. 9A)** edge of the isthmocele from the apex to the cervical outer orifice after a careful evaluation of pouch depth with the loop electrode.

After having flattered the proximal edge, the procedure goes on with the resection of the fibrotic tissue of the distal margin (step 2) of the niche **(Fig. 9B)** and ends completely removing the inflamed tissue of all cervical canal walls around the proximal and distal margin at 360° thus completing the endocervical ablation.[9]

Depending on the electrosurgical unit, a high-frequency 90° angled circular loop electrode is used with a pure cut current at a power setting of 100 watts/s for monopolar energy and with maximum cutting effect for bipolar energy. A high-frequency angled ball electrode is then used to obtain focused vaporization of all residual inflamed tissue still present on the niche surface/ceiling (step 3) **(Fig. 9C)**.

Before removing the resectoscope, the reduction of the inflow and pressure of the distending medium helps to identify any endocervical vessels bleeding. A focused coagulation is obtained with a high-frequency angled ball electrode (step 4) and is used to prevent any postprocedure bleeding.

A variety of approaches including laparotomy, laparoscopy, hysteroscopy, vaginal repair, and various other combined techniques have been used, but the outcomes were not significantly different among the various procedures.[10]

Hysteroscopic isthmoplaty, restoring the continuity of the cervical canal **(Figs. 10A and B)** has been generally shown to be effective for symptom relief and fertility improvement and to be easy managed in day surgery setting.[11]

Hysteroscopic radical isthmoplaty (Channel-like 360°) using 15–16-Fr resectoscope has been shown to be minimally invasive with low morbidity. Complications such as cervical laceration or false passage due to Hegar dilatation are avoided with vaginoscopic approach. Moreover, complications such as uterine perforation, bladder injury during hysteroscopic procedure have never been described.[12]

Nevertheless, several authors are fully aware of this possibility and recommended laparoscopic or vaginal repair when RMT is between 2 and 3.5 mm.[13]

Since RMT minimum size has been arbitrarily considered a key parameter in determining the choice of surgical technique and outcomes, symptom relief, increase RMT, fertility improvement, and prevention of uterine rupture are not significantly different among the various procedures.[14]

The final decision is based on the skill of the surgeon and his ability to use one or other surgical approaches in which the operator is more trained and confident.

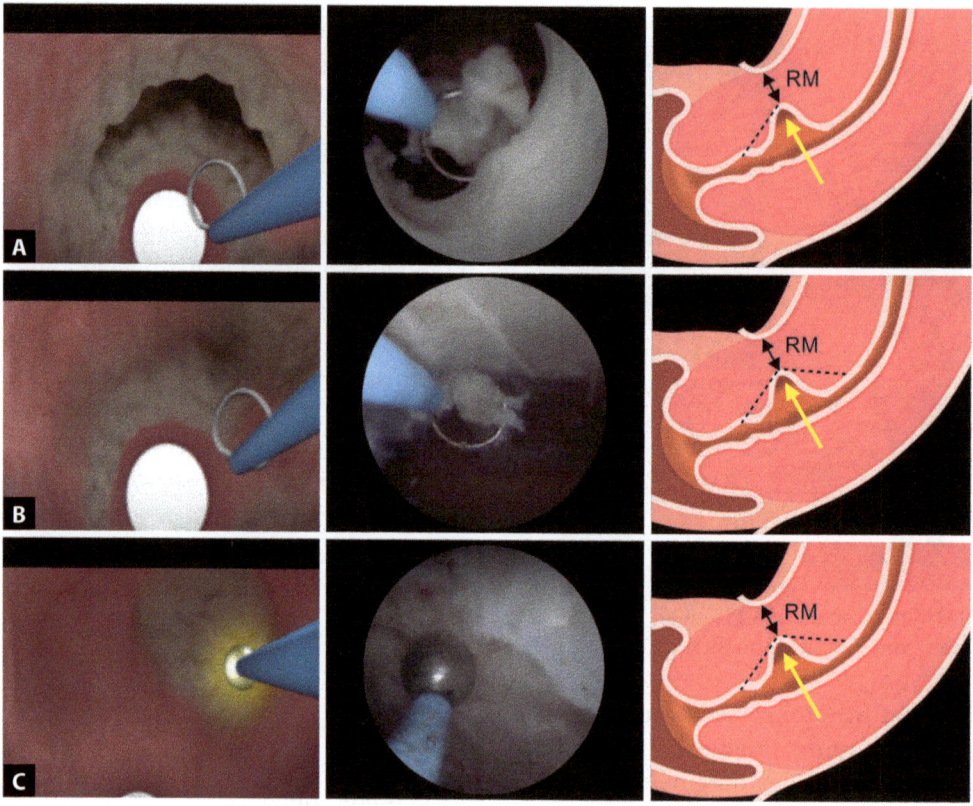

Figs. 9A to C: Channel-like resectoscopic treatment of CSD. (A) First step: Resection of the fibrotic tissue of the proximal/inferior part; (B) Second step: Resection of the fibrotic tissue of the distal/superior part; (C) Third step: Superficially vaporization of niche surface (ceiling) with a roller ball electrode. (CSD: cesarean scar defect)

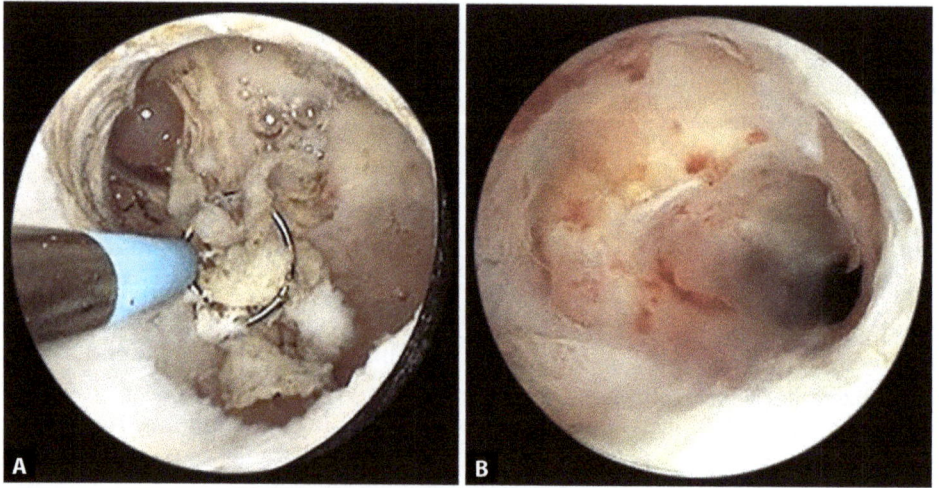

Figs. 10A and B: Hysteroscopic isthmocele appearance (A) during resection of fibrotic tissue and (B) after 6-month follow-up.

■ CONCLUSION

Hysteroscopic 360° channel-like resection:
- Decreases the size of CSD (height, transverse diameter, and volume)
- Increases RMT
- Re-establishes a channel shape of the cervical canal
- Restores the normal flow of menstrual blood through the cervix

- Removes inflamed tissue of all cervical canal walls around the proximal and distal margin
- Facilitates the re-epithelialization of the cervical canal walls by a paraphysiological endocervical epithelium
- Improves postmenstrual symptoms (spotting, dark red or brown discharge), pain and cervical mucus quality
- Restores fertility.

REFERENCES

1. Tsuji S, Nobuta Y, Hanada T, Takebayashi A, Inatomi A, Takahashi A, et al. Prevalence, definition, and etiology of cesarean scar defect and treatment of cesarean scar disorder: A narrative review. Reprod Med Biol. 2023;22:e12532.
2. Bij de Vaate AJ, Linskens IH, van derVoet LF, Twisk JW, Brölmann HA, Huirne JA. Reproducibility of three-dimensional ultrasound for the measurement of a niche in a cesarean scar and assessment of its shape. Eur J Obstet Gynecol Reprod Biol. 2015;188:39-44.
3. Kulshrestha V, Agarwal N, Kachhawa G. Post-caesarean Niche (Isthmocele) in uterine scar: an update. J Obstet Gynaecol India. 2020;70(6):440-6.
4. Jordans IPM, de Leeuw RA, Stegwee SI, Amso NN, Barri-Soldevila PN, van den Bosch T, et al. Sonographic examination of uterine isthmocele in non-pregnant women: a modified Delphi procedure. Ultrasound Obstet Gynecol. 2019;53:107-15.
5. Fabres C, Arriagada P, Fernandez C, Mackenna A, Zegers F, Fernández E. Surgical treatment and follow-up of women with intermenstrual bleeding due to cesarean section scar defect. J Minim Invasive Gynecol. 2005;12(1):25-8.
6. Gubbini G, Casadio P, Marra E. Resectoscopic correction of the "isthmocele" in women with postmenstrual abnormal uterine bleeding and secondary infertility. J Minim Invasive Gynecol. 2008;15(2):172-5.
7. Di Spiezio Sardo A, Zizolfi B, Calagna G, Giampaolino P, Paolella F, Bifulco G. Hysteroscopic isthmoplasty: step by step technique. J Minim Invasive Gynecol. 2018;25(2):338-9.
8. Casadio P, Gubbini G, Franchini M, Morra C, Talamo MR, Magnarelli G, et al. Comparison of hysteroscopic cesarean scar defect repair with 26 Fr resectoscope and 16 Fr mini-resectoscope: a prospective pilot study. J Minim Invasive Gynecol. 2021;28(2):314-9.
9. Casadio P, Gubbini G, Morra C, Franchini M, Paradisi R, Seracchioli R. Channel-like 360° isthmocele treatment with a 16 F mini-resectoscope: a step-by-step technique. J Minim Invasive Gynecol. 2019;26(7):1229-30.
10. Donnez O. Cesarean scar disorder: Management and repair. Best Pract Res Clin Obstet Gynaecol. 2023;90:102398.
11. Dominguez JA, Alonso Pacheco L, Moratalla E, Carugno JA, Carrera M, Perez-Milan F, et al. Diagnosis and management of isthmocele (Cesarean scar defect): a SWOT analysis. Ultrasound Obstet Gynecol. 2023;62(3):336-44.
12. Giampietro G, Casadio P, Franchini M, Florio P. Regarding "optimal timing and recommended route of delivery after hysteroscopic management of isthmocele? A consensus statement from the global congress on hysteroscopy scientific committee". J Minim Invasive Gynecol. 2018; 25(6):1111-2.
13. Laganà AS, Pacheco LA, Tinelli A, Haimovich S, Carugno J, Ghezzi F, Global Congress on Hysteroscopy Scientific Committee. Optimal timing and recommended route of delivery after hysteroscopic management of isthmocele? A consensus statement from the Global Congress on Hysteroscopy Scientific Committee. J Minim Invasive Gynecol. 2018;25(4):558.
14. Casadio P, Raffone A, Alletto A, Filipponi F, Raimondo D, Arena A, et al. Postoperative morphologic changes of the isthmocele and clinical impact in patients treated by channel-like (360°) hysteroscopic technique. Int J Gynaecol Obstet. 2022;160:326-33.

Proximal Tubal Cannulation, Making Simplified

Chapter 12

Mykhailo V Medvediev

■ INTRODUCTION

The first documented effort to insert instruments through the vagina to access the tubal lumen via the uterotubal ostium (UTO) is credited to Tyler Smith in 1849. 6 years later, in 1856, Gardner outlined a technique for the transvaginal insertion of incrementally sized probes. By 1970, a 1-mm diameter fibroscope was employed to inspect the tubal lumen; however, due to inadequate lighting and technical challenges, thorough examination was problematic. Today, intraluminal tubal endoscopy can be carried out through either a transvaginal route, known as falloscopy, or a transabdominal route, referred to as salpingoscopy.[1]

In this chapter, our focus will be squarely on proximal tubal cannulation (PTC), a specialized procedure aimed at addressing proximal tubal occlusions (PTOs). This technique is particularly relevant for cases where the blockage occurs near the uterotubal junction, and it is especially crucial when the remainder of the pelvic anatomy presents as normal.[2]

■ ETIOLOGY OF PROXIMAL TUBAL OCCLUSION

The etiology of PTO is multifactorial, often involving infection, prior surgical interventions, and sometimes congenital anomalies.

Fallopian tube diseases such as tubal blockages, pelvic inflammatory disease (PID), or tubal scarring can significantly contribute to infertility rates among women. The reported range of 11–67% in the incidence of tubal factors causing infertility is quite broad, mainly due to differences in study populations, diagnostic criteria, and testing methods.[3]

Between 10 and 25% of tubal factor infertility cases may be attributed to a specific condition known as PTO. This condition is especially noteworthy because it occurs even when the rest of the pelvic anatomy appears to be normal. Unlike other types of tubal blockages, proximal occlusion affects the segment of the fallopian tube closest to the uterus, which can complicate both diagnosis and treatment.[4]

Proximal tubal occlusion refers to the blockage of the proximal section of the fallopian tube, adjacent to the uterine wall. It is a significant cause of infertility in women. Understanding its etiology is crucial for targeted treatment and potentially preventing the condition.

Causes:
- Pelvic inflammatory disease and infections, such as chlamydia and gonorrhea, which can cause scarring and blockage
- *Endometriosis:* Presence of endometrial tissue outside the uterus can cause adhesions and blockages
- *Previous tubal surgery:* Adhesions formed postsurgery may cause occlusion.
- *Congenital anomalies:* Malformations of the fallopian tube present from birth can lead to blockages.
- *Ectopic pregnancy:* Past ectopic pregnancies can cause scarring and obstruction.
- *Iatrogenic causes:* Blockage due to medical procedures such as hysterosalpingogram or other uterine procedures.
- *Salpingitis isthmica nodosa (SIN):* This is a specific pathological condition that affects the fallopian tubes, more commonly at the isthmus, the narrower, muscle-rich segment near the uterine end. It is characterized by the presence of diverticula, or nodular thickenings, that form because of chronic inflammation. These nodules can obstruct the tube, thereby affecting fertility, or may even predispose the patient to ectopic pregnancies. Diagnosis often involves imaging techniques such as hysterosalpingography (HSG) or more invasive

methods such as laparoscopy for direct visualization of the tubal structures. It is worth noting that SIN is sometimes an incidental finding during investigations for infertility or tubal disease.[5] The pathology of SIN involves thickening of the muscular layer of the tube and formation of microscopic diverticula that can extend into the lumen, causing partial or complete blockage. The exact etiology is not well-understood, but it may include inflammatory factors and possibly an aberrant response to prior infections.[6]

■ CLINICAL PRESENTATION

Patients may be asymptomatic or present with symptoms of chronic pelvic pain, infertility, or history of ectopic pregnancy. The disease often coexists with other gynecological disorders such as endometriosis and pelvic inflammatory disease.

Accurate diagnosis is pivotal for targeted treatment approaches, such as PTC, to restore fertility.

■ DIAGNOSIS AND PLANNING

Preoperative preparation:
- *Patient counseling:* Thoroughly discuss the risks and benefits of the procedure, and obtain informed consent.
- *Imaging:* Conduct diagnostic tests like hysterosalpingography or laparoscopy to confirm the site of the tubal blockage.
- *Antibiotic prophylaxis:* Administer prophylactic antibiotics to minimize infection risk.
- The patient is generally scheduled for examination within the 5th–11th day of her menstrual cycle, specifically during the follicular phase, prior to ovulation.

Diagnostic tools for proximal tubal occlusion assessment:
- Hysterosalpingogram (HSG)
- Saline sonohysterography
- Laparoscopy

Before suggesting retrograde tubular canalization, alternative techniques that provide more stable results should be considered. Such methods include in vitro fertilization (IVF).

In addition, as an alternative to PCT resection of the fallopian tube with further reimplantation can be considered.

Indications for PTC:
- Infertility due to proximal tubal occlusion
- Failure of previous conventional treatments
- Prior to in vitro fertilization for tubal factor infertility (in case of patient's desire to try this option first).

Risks and complications of PTC:
- Perforation of the tube
- Infection
- Allergic reactions to contrast
- Bleeding and hematoma
Overall, the complication rate does not exceed 1–2%.[2]

Outcome assessment:
- Success rate varies, but generally around 60–70%[7,8]
- Subsequent pregnancy outcomes are influenced by various factors including maternal age, sperm quality, and overall health; generally, success rates range from 30 to 50%.[7-9]
- The chance of a woman having an ectopic pregnancy is 4%.[9]

■ OPERATIVE TIPS

Equipment

- *Hysteroscope:* For visualization of the uterine cavity, we typically employ a 5 mm hysteroscope with a 30-degree lens, equipped with both inflow and outflow channels as well as an instrumental channel.
- *Microcatheter and guidewire:* For tubal cannulation, we usually utilize modified Novy cornual cannulation **(Figs. 1 to 4)**
- *Fluoroscopy unit:* For real-time X-ray guidance (optional).

Operative Steps

- *Access the uterine cavity:* Insert a hysteroscope into the uterine cavity for initial visualization.
- *Identify the tubal ostia:* Locate the tubal openings within the uterine cavity.

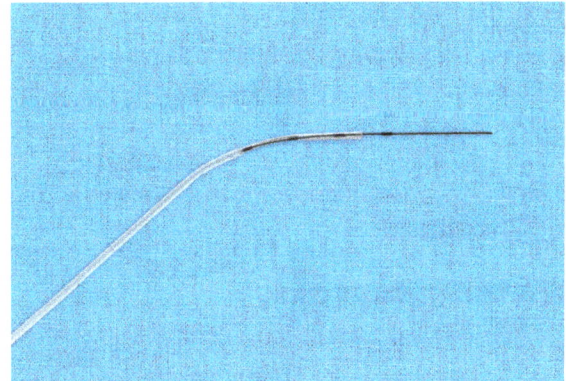

Fig. 1: Modified Novy cornual cannulation set.[10]

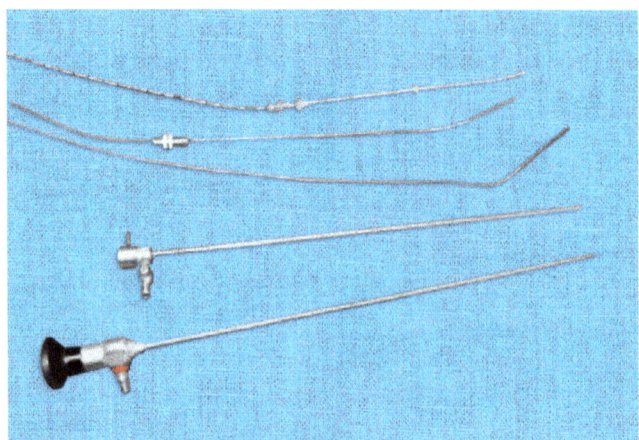

Fig. 2: A complete set of tubal cannulation instruments.[8]

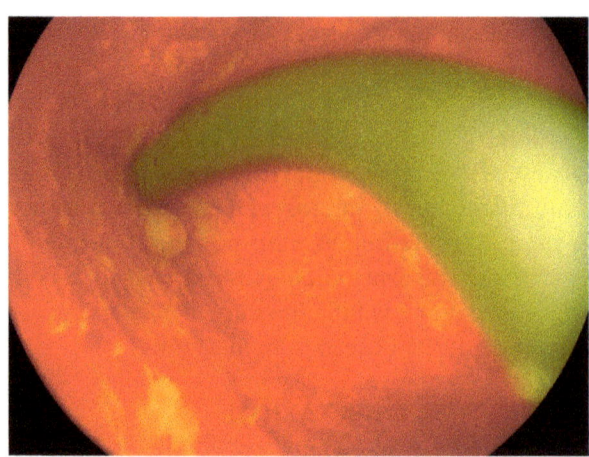

Fig. 4: Hysteroscopic visualization of tubal cannulation featuring the Novy catheter inserted into the left tubal ostium.[7]

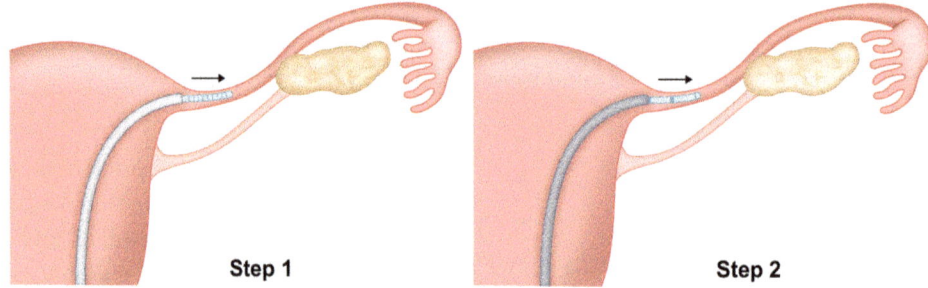

Fig. 3: Schematic representation of catheter insertion with guidewire, overcoming the site of occlusion, and lavage of the tubal lumen with saline solution.[10]

- *Insert microcatheter:* Advance the microcatheter through the hysteroscope toward the identified tubal ostium.
- *Guidewire introduction:* Introduce a guidewire through the microcatheter and navigate it toward the site of obstruction under real-time imaging guidance, if available.
- *Overcome the obstruction:* Gently push the guidewire forward to penetrate the blockage. If resistance is met, do not force the wire as it could cause tubal damage.
- *Confirm placement:* Once past the obstruction, confirm the placement by injecting a contrast medium if fluoroscopy is used **(Figs. 5A to E)**.
- *Remove instruments:* After confirmation, carefully retract the guidewire and microcatheter.
- *End the procedure:* Remove the hysteroscope and finish the procedure.

POSTOPERATIVE CARE

- *Surveillance for adverse outcomes*: Maintain vigilance for clinical indicators of infection or fallopian tube damage.
- *Postprocedure imaging*: Arrange for subsequent hysterosalpingography to verify the success of the cannulation technique.
- *Postintervention fertility evaluation*: Conduct a comprehensive fertility assessment following an adequate time interval postprocedure.

TIPS AND CAUTIONS

- Always advance instruments gently to minimize trauma to the fallopian tubes.
- Using real-time imaging, like fluoroscopy, can enhance the success rate.
- Do not force the guidewire if resistance is felt; instead, reassess the situation.

CONCLUSION

Proximal tubal cannulation is a delicate, skill-demanding procedure that can provide substantial benefits in treating infertility due to proximal tubal occlusion. Following these operative tips and best practices can increase the chances of a successful outcome.

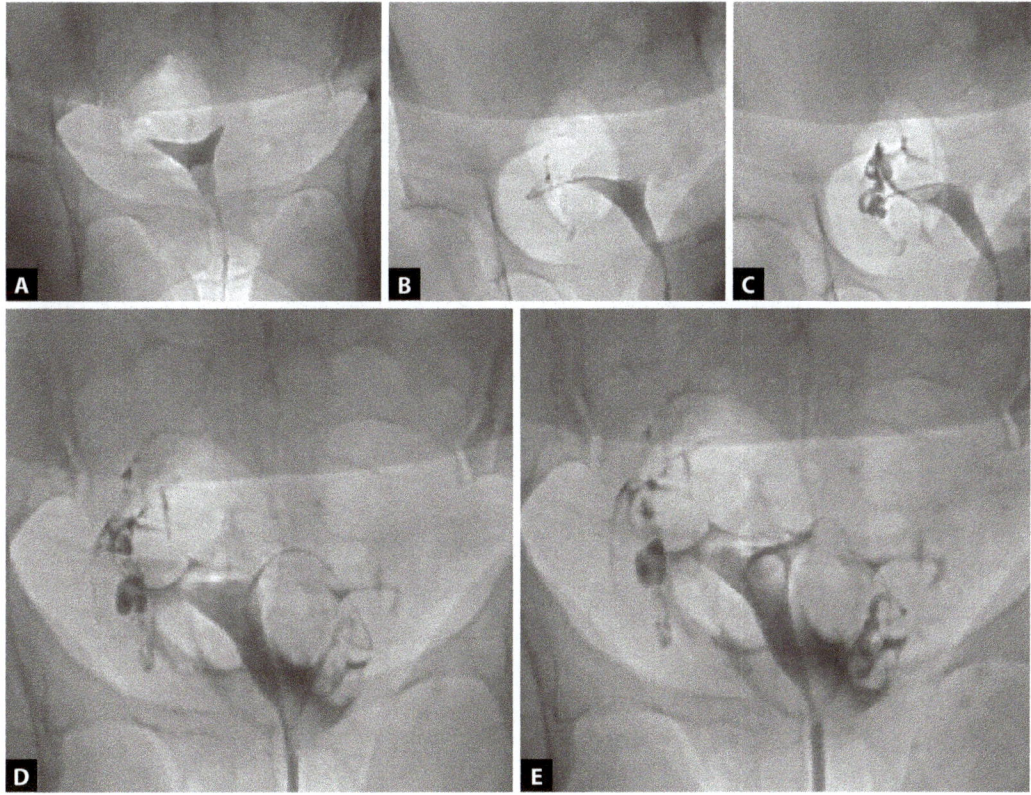

Figs. 5A to E: The hysterosalpingogram (HSG) series demonstrates various stages of tubal evaluation:[2] (A) Displays bilateral tubal occlusion, indicating both tubes are blocked; (B) Reveals the presence of a guidewire in the proximal portion of the right fallopian tube, signifying an attempt to navigate the occlusion; (C) Depicts a patent right fallopian tube, suggesting successful recanalization or that the obstruction has been surpassed; (D) Exhibits the guidewire inserted into the fallopian tube, confirming its intraluminal position; (E) Illustrates the patency of the left fallopian tube, indicating that it is open and unobstructed.

REFERENCES

1. El-Mowafi Diaa M, Nkele Ndeki N. Management of tubal obstructions. Surg Technol Int. 2005;14:199-212.
2. Anne R. Fallopian tube recanalization for the management of infertility. CVIR Endovasc. 2023;6(1):13.
3. Carson SA, Kallen AN. Diagnosis and Management of Infertility: A Review. JAMA. 2021;326(1):65-76.
4. Al-Omari MH, Obeidat N, Elheis M, Khasawneh RA, Gharaibeh MM. Factors affecting pregnancy rate following fallopian tube recanalization in women with proximal fallopian tube obstruction. J Clin Med. 2018;7(5):110.
5. Practice Committee of the American Society for Reproductive Medicine. Practice Committee of the American Society for Reproductive Medicine. Committee opinion: role of tubal surgery in the era of assisted reproductive technology. Fertil Steril. 2012;97(3):539-45.
6. David B, Tobler Kyle J. Salpingitis Isthmica Nodosa. StatPearls. Treasure Island (FL): StatPearls Publishing; 2023.
7. Martin K, Brown Emma C, Frishman Gary N, May-Tal SC. Fluoroscopically-guided hysteroscopic tubal cannulation: A Procedure for Proximal Tubal Obstruction. JSLS. 2022;26(4):e2022.00047.
8. Soliman AT, Salem HA. Evaluation of hysteroscopic tubal cannulation under laparoscopic control versus intracytoplasmic sperm injection in cases with proximal tubal obstruction. J Evidence-Based Women's Health J Soc. 2013;3(3):147.
9. De Silva PM, Chu JJ, Gallos ID, Vidyasagar AT, Robinson L, Coomarasamy A. Fallopian tube catheterization in the treatment of proximal tubal obstruction: a systematic review and meta-analysis. Hum Reprod. 2017;32(4):836-52.
10. Cook Medical. Modified Novy Cornual Cannulation Set. [online] Available from: https://www.cookmedical.com/products/wh_ncs_webds/. [Last accessed November, 2023].

Hysteroscopy in Retained Products of Conception

Chapter 13

Milind A Telang, Jui Telang

INTRODUCTION

Hysteroscopy is the eye of the gynecologist in the endometrial cavity. With increase in cases of medical termination of pregnancy with mifepristone and misoprostol combination the cases of retained products are increasing in day-to-day practice.

INCIDENCE

Incidence is 0.5–1% of all surgical abortions in first trimester and increases to 6% in second trimester. Incidence is higher in medical abortions. About 1% of all term pregnancies are complicated by persistence of retained trophoblastic tissue.

SEQUELAE

- Bleeding
- Endometritis
- Intrauterine adhesions (IUAs)
- Secondary infertility.

PATHOGENESIS

Eastman and Hellman theory: Decidua formation is less in cornua/fundal/lower uterine segment. In case of implantation in these areas, chorionic villi get attached to myometrium resulting in retention.

Ranney theory: Direct relationship of thickness and tone in different areas of myometrium with existence of retained products. Fundal and uterotubal areas are relatively atonic after second stage.

DIAGNOSIS

Limited value of β-hCG (human chorionic gonadotropin) estimation. Retained products can maintain endocrine activity at very low levels of hCG.

First-line diagnostic test is transvaginal sonography. An inhomogeneous intracavitary hyperechoic focal or scattered mass is suggestive. Color Doppler is useful to identify vascular variant with increasing neovascularity going up to the myometrium.

Correlation of Ultrasonography and Hysteroscopy

The Gutenberg classification by Luis Alonso et al.[1] is a useful guide on sonography and can be correlated with hysteroscopic images **(Table 1)**.

Hysteroscopy is gold standard for diagnosis of endometrial cavity pathologies and so is the procedure of choice in diagnosis and treating of retained products (see-and-treat).[2] In cases of heavy bleeding, the option is to stop or decrease the bleeding and then proceed.

Traditionally D and C is the most common intervention.

According to the Malaga declaration of 2022, blind procedures in intrauterine cavity should be avoided. The chance of IUAs after one D and C is 16% and goes up to 32% after two. In addition, the risk of anesthesia, blind

TABLE 1: Correlation of ultrasonography (USG) and hysteroscopy.

	USG	Hysteroscopy
Type 0	Avascular hyperechogenic	White mass with no identifiable structure
Type 1	Different grades of echogenicity with minimal vascularity	Well defined/avascular. Chorionic villi seen
Type 2	Hypervascularized mass hyperechoic	Well-defined well-vascularized chorionic villi with yellow discoloration
Type 3	Hypervascularized mass with vascularized myometrium	Resembles A-V malformation

dilatation, and increased chances of perforation are associated with D and C.

Focal retained products of conception (RPOC) are missed by D and C. According to Cohen SB et al., residual tissue after D and C is 20.8%.

Goldenberg in 1997 first reported resectoscopy for selective removal of RPOC. Under direct vision with cutting loop, successful removal of RPOC was achieved. No injury to neighboring endometrium prevented formation of IUA.

The loop of electrode can be used to dissect the RPOC without current. In Type 0 and 1, resectoscopic loop can be used as cold curette. In Type 2, electrocautery is essential to fulgurate the site of implantation.

With the advent of 15-Fr mini-resectoscope, the removal of RPOC can be done in outpatient setting with conscious sedation and no dilatation.

The Bettocchi 5 or Bettocchi 4 hysteroscopes with crocodile forceps 5 Fr can be used in office. The technique is to detach the RPOC from the bed by repeatedly opening and closing the jaws of the grasper. Bipolar needle 5 Fr can be used to coagulate bleeding vessel.

The mechanical tissue retrieval system (mHTR) 15 Fr and 17 Fr can be used in office without any form of anesthesia and premedication for removal of RPOC **(Fig. 1)**. Under vision in one insertion of the blade without damage to the normal endometrium. All the material is collected in canister for histopathology. No chances of IUAs. Fear of bleeding is more theoretical as once pressure reduced, the myometrium contracts and subdues the bleeding.

Post-treatment, the pregnancy rates of 50–88% depending on technique used.

The advantages of hysteroscopy:
- Direct visualization
- Complete and selective removal without damaging neighboring endometrium
- Specimen for histopathology

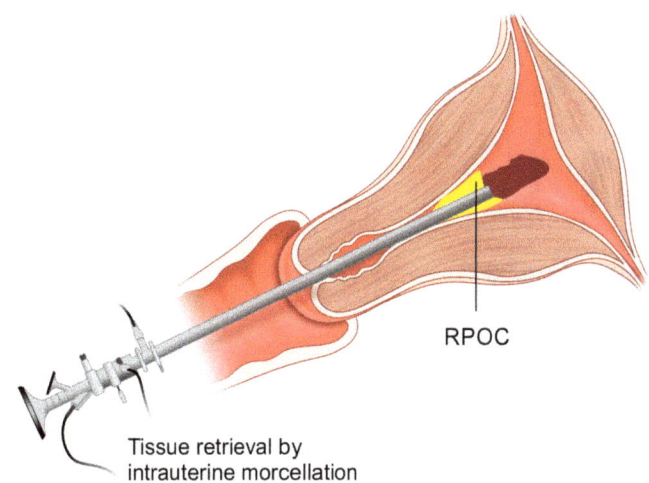

Fig. 1: Mechanical tissue retrieval system. (RPOC: retained products of conception)

- Chances of IUAs minimal
- Early conception

This definitely makes it the treatment of choice for retained products (RPOC).

CONCLUSION

In today's era of "SEE & TREAT" blind procedures must be avoided. Hysteroscopic removal of retained products is the method of choice and removal by tissue retrieval system is ideal.

REFERENCES

1. Alonso L, Pacheco L, Pascual N. Atlas of Hysteroscopy. Springer International Publishing AG A. Tinelli, et al (Eds), Hysteroscopy; 2018.
2. Smorgick N, Levinsohn-Tavor O, Ben-Ami I, Maymon R, Pansky M, Vaknin Z. Hysteroscopic removal of retained products of conception following first trimester medical abortion. Gynecol Minim Invasive Ther. 2017;6(4):183-5.

14 Misplaced Foreign Bodies in the Uterine Cavity

Pankaj Mate

INTRODUCTION

Foreign bodies in the uterine cavity can be encountered in all age groups and may cause offensive vaginal discharge, pain in abdomen, chronic pelvic pain, pelvic inflammatory disease (PID), and infertility.

Inside the uterus, retained products of conception, tip of curette, laminaria tent, nonabsorbable suture material, CuT, and Lippes loop **(Fig. 1)** have been reported. In one rare case, infant feeding tube kept in uterus and both fallopian tubes post tubal recanalization for patency was removed (which was supposed to be removed hysteroscopically after operation).

CAUSES OF MISPLACED FOREIGN BODIES

There are several causes that can lead to foreign bodies becoming lodged in the uterine cavity. Some of the common causes include:

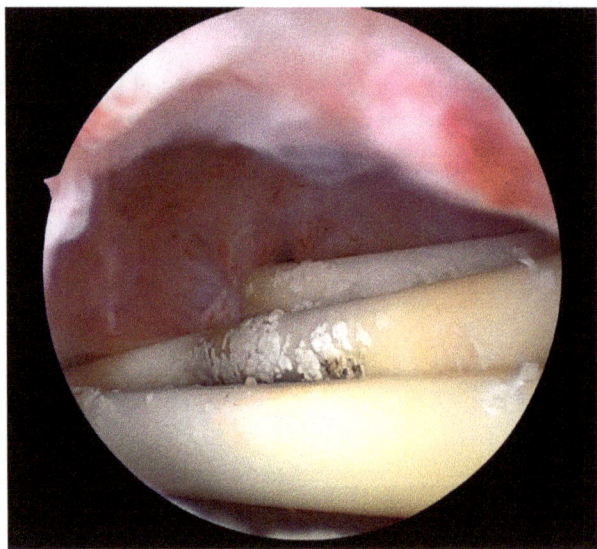

Fig. 1: Misplaced Lippes loop in uterine cavity.

- *Intrauterine devices (IUDs):* IUDs are a popular form of contraception, but there can be instances where they may become displaced or migrate from their original position within the uterus.
- *Surgical instruments:* During certain medical procedures, such as dilation and curettage (D and C) or hysteroscopy, small instruments may inadvertently break and remain in the uterus.
- *Accidental insertion:* Foreign bodies can sometimes be accidentally inserted into the uterine cavity, such as tampons or contraceptive devices.

CLINICAL PRESENTATION

The presence of a misplaced foreign body in the uterine cavity may lead to various signs and symptoms. These can include:
- Abnormal vaginal bleeding or discharge
- Pelvic pain or discomfort
- Infertility or recurrent miscarriages
- Vaginal infections or recurrent urinary tract infections
- Unexplained fever or PID.

Intrauterine Devices

Intrauterine contraceptive device (IUCD) is a popular method of long-term reversible contraception with failure rate of less than one per 100 women-years. The device is located within the endometrial cavity **(Fig. 2)** or cervical canal **(Fig. 3)** in 95% of the cases.[1] Missing IUCD strings **(Fig. 4)** are observed in about 5% of the users.[2]

The differential diagnosis of missing IUCD strings includes unnoticed expulsion, misplacement outside the uterine cavity, broken or severed IUCD strings, and string retraction into the cervical canal or endometrial cavity due to rotation of the device **(Fig. 5)**.

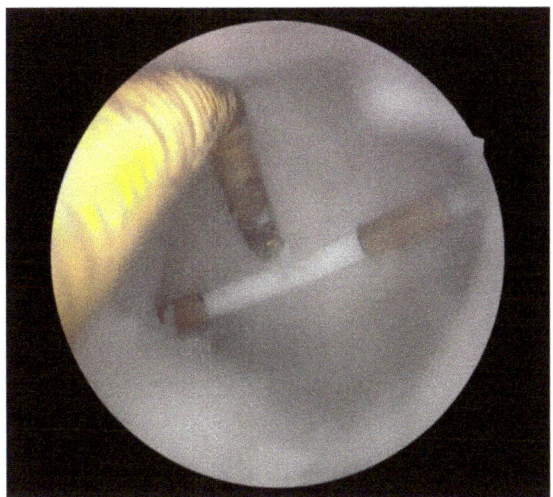

Fig. 2: Intrauterine contraceptive device in situ.

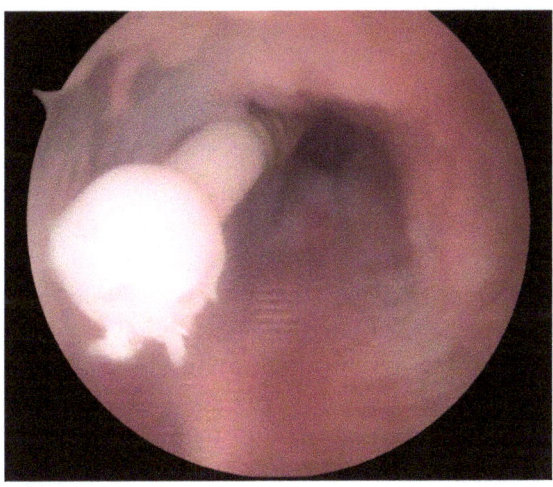

Fig. 3: Intrauterine contraceptive device in cervical canal.

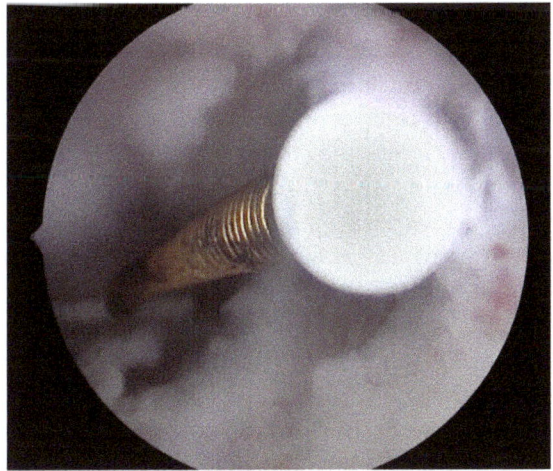

Fig. 4: Intrauterine contraceptive device with missing string.

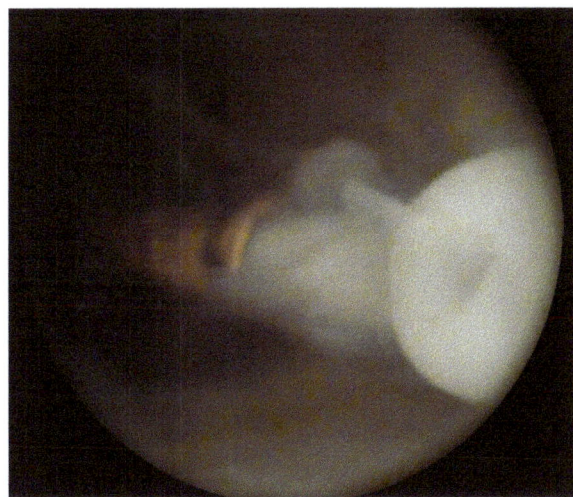

Fig. 5: String folded back in to the uterine cavity.

However, in a few cases, it can perforate the uterus and migrate into adjoining structures. Sites of migration are usually within pelvis or in omentum but at times the device may migrate far into upper abdomen. Various factors such as spontaneous expulsion, fragmentation of IUCD, uterine contractions, and incidental pregnancy may cause secondary displacement of IUCD.

Perforation may be asymptomatic or symptomatic. Though rare but misplaced IUCDs may cause dangerous complications like bowel and bladder perforation. Even if asymptomatic, all misplaced IUCDs lying outside the uterus should be retrieved through laparoscopy or laparotomy to avoid complications such as adhesions, fistula formation, and intestinal obstruction.

Other Foreign Bodies

Laminaria tent: Laminaria is a small rod of hydroscopic dehydrated seaweed used for cervical dilatation in various obstetrical and gynecological procedures. Complications of laminaria use are rare, but may include infection, anaphylaxis, retention, and fragmentation. Several case reports and a series of 22 patients with complications of laminaria in which extraction was difficult using customary measures (like vacuum aspiration, sharp curettage, and ultrasound forceps extraction) have been reported.[3]

Endometrial osseous metaplasia—is a rare pathological condition with mature bone in the endometrium and can be a cause for menorrhagia and infertility as bone in the endometrium acts like intrauterine contraceptive device. Osseous metaplasia **(Fig. 6)** occurs in approximately 0.3 per 10,000 women.[4]

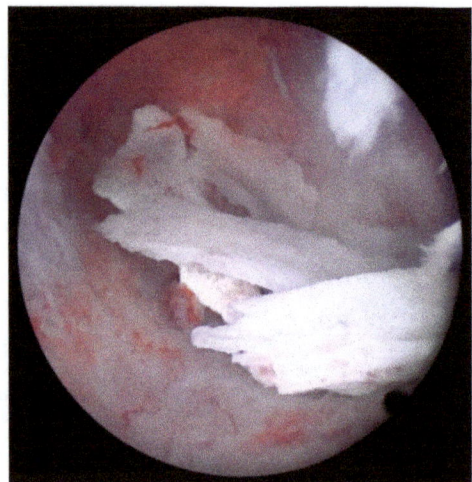

Fig. 6: Bone fragments in osseous metaplasia.

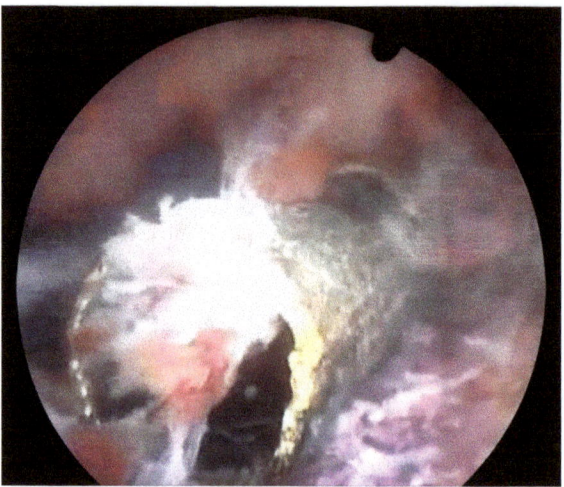

Fig. 8: Broken metal cannula tip during D and E.

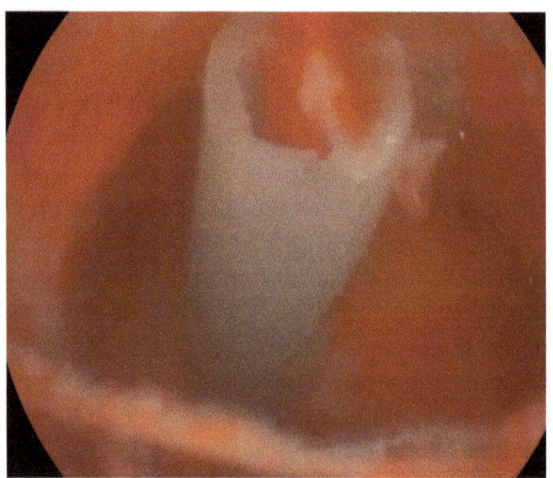

Fig. 7: Broken Karman cannula tip.

Although the etiology of this rare condition is unknown, the most widely accepted hypothesis is that ossification is related to retained fetal bones, following abortion suggesting endochondral ossification. It also may be related to transformation of mesenchymal tissue to osseous tissue in response to inflammation and the reparative process induced by abortion. It is an endogenous non-neoplastic pathological condition as no tissue reaction is found in the endometrial tissue and the endometrium shows normal regular cyclical changes.[5]

A broken suction cannula tip during medical termination of pregnancy: The breaking of the tip of a suction cannula—plastic (**Fig. 7**) or metal (**Fig. 8**), while performing a suction evacuation procedure is a rare complication.

Suture Material

Obstetricians usually use absorbable sutures to close hysterotomy in the cesarean section.[6] If the sutures used during cesarean section or hysterotomy undergo inappropriate hydrolysis and absorption, the retained intrauterine sutures may cause intrauterine inflammations with subsequent abnormal uterine bleeding (AUB) and/or infertility.

The retained intrauterine sutures may interfere with sperm transport and implantation and act as a foreign body with subsequent intrauterine inflammation and infertility.

Using a nonabsorbable suture for hysterotomy closure may lead to foreign body reactions.

DIAGNOSIS

Detailed history and clinical examination are very much essential for diagnosis and prevention of morbidity and mortality resulting from complications.

To accurately diagnose a misplaced foreign body in the uterine cavity, several diagnostic methods may be utilized. These include:
- *Pelvic examination*: Nonvisualization of IUCD strings is suggestive of misplaced device. A thorough examination of the pelvic region may reveal any abnormalities or signs of infection.
- *Ultrasound*: Transvaginal ultrasound can provide detailed images of the uterine cavity and in localizing the misplaced IUCD accurately (**Fig. 9**). This is essential for planning the appropriate intervention to retrieve the device.

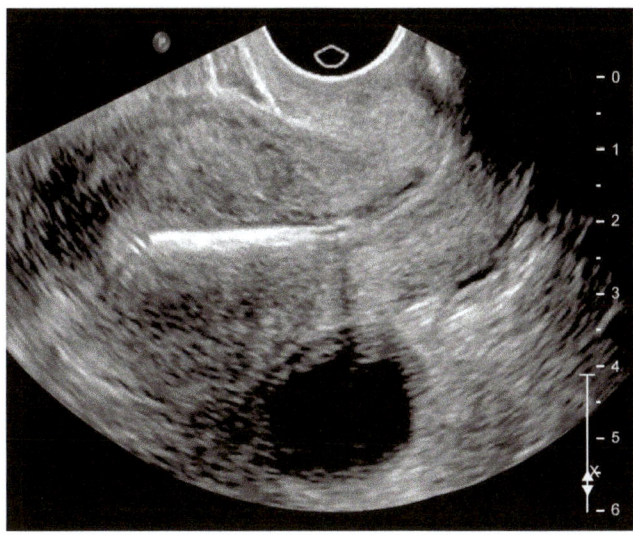

Fig. 9: In situ intrauterine contraceptive device on ultrasound.

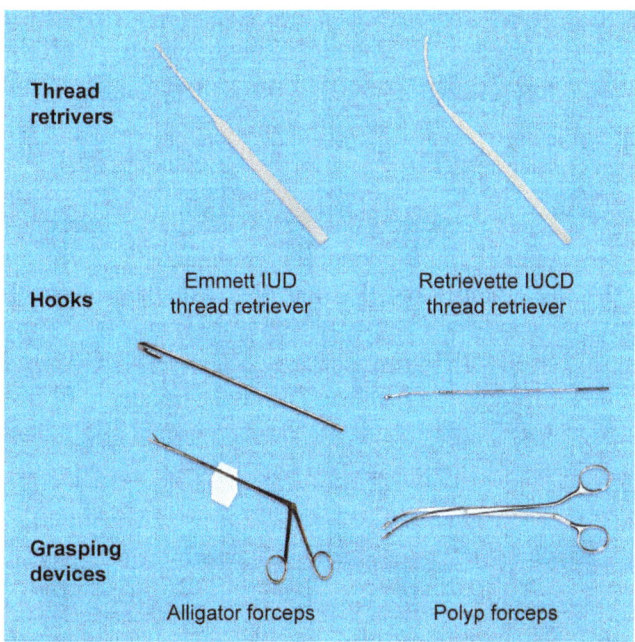

Fig. 10: Intrauterine contraceptive retrieval devices.
(IUCD: intrauterine contraceptive device; IUD: intrauterine device)

- Hysteroscopy—is gold standard allowing direct visualization of the uterine cavity and the retrieval of any foreign bodies.

■ TREATMENT OPTIONS

The management of foreign bodies in the uterine cavity depends on several factors, including the type and location of the foreign body, patient's symptoms, and the presence of any associated complications.

The treatment of misplaced foreign bodies in the uterine cavity aims to remove the foreign body and address any associated complications. The treatment options may include:

- *Manual removal:* In some cases, a misplaced foreign body with strings in cervical canal or in uterine cavity can be manually removed by a healthcare professional during a pelvic examination. IUCD in cervical canal can be removed with the help of long artery forceps. Thread retrievers are available (three types of thread retrievers are described: the Mi-Mark helix, the Emmett IUC retrieval device, and the Retrievette IUCD retrieval device) and are inserted into the cervix using a clockwise twisting motion during both entrance into the uterine cavity and exit out the cervix **(Fig. 10)**.

  Verma et al. reported their experience with ultrasound-guided removal of retained IUDs, as safe and cost-effective, and it could be performed in an office setting.[7]

- *Hysteroscopic removal:* If the foreign body is lodged deep within the uterine cavity **(Fig. 11)** or arm of IUCD

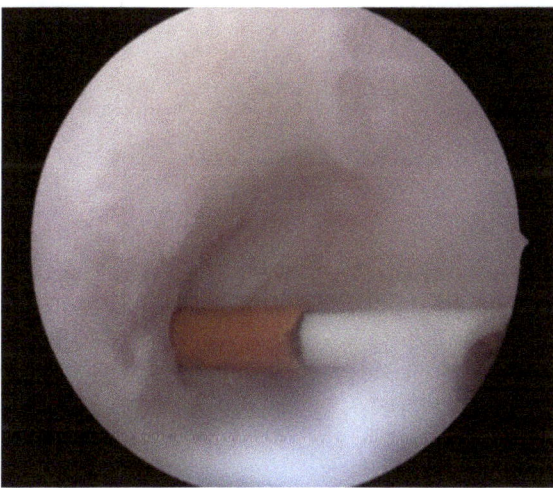

Fig. 11: Embedded CuT arm in to the uterine lateral wall.

is broken **(Fig. 12)** or cannot be easily retrieved, a hysteroscopy may be performed. Hysteroscopy is the preferred method in management of misplaced foreign body in uterine cavity. It allows direct visualization of the uterine cavity, facilitating the removal of the foreign body.

- Under general anesthesia, the patient is placed in the lithotomy position, cleaned, and draped. Cusco's speculum introduced, and the cervix was visualized, which is held using the vulsellum.

- If needed dilatation of the cervix can be performed using Hegar's dilator to gain entry into the uterus.
- Normal saline is used as a distension media. The outflow track of the hysteroscope can be intermittently opened due to which the vision was not hampered.
- The operative hysteroscopy sheath is introduced through the endocervical canal.
- Frequently IUCD string or the distal end of the device is visible (*see* **Figs. 3 and 4**).
- Using a hysteroscopic grasping forceps introduced through the working channel, the string or the distal end of the IUCD can be grasped and pulled out the uterine cavity (**Figs. 13 and 14**).
- In case of broken tip of suction cannula, the hysteroscopic grasper would be too small to catch heavy and large broken plastic/metal tip (**Figs. 15 and 16**). The hysteroscopic grasper would also break while trying to hold a larger and heavier object like the metal tip. The laparoscopic 5-mm tenaculum can be passed alongside the hysteroscope with which the tip could be removed vertically with the least diameter.
- Nowadays, hysteroscopic or resectoscopic operation is preferred over dilatation and curettage for the removal of osseous tissue from the uterus (**Figs. 17 and 18**). Especially, the ultrasound-guided hysteroscopy may be applied to facilitate removal of osseous tissue.

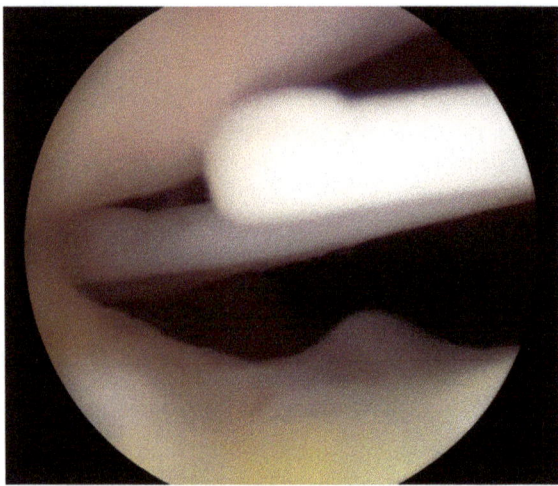

Fig. 12: Misplaced broken arm of multiload CuT.

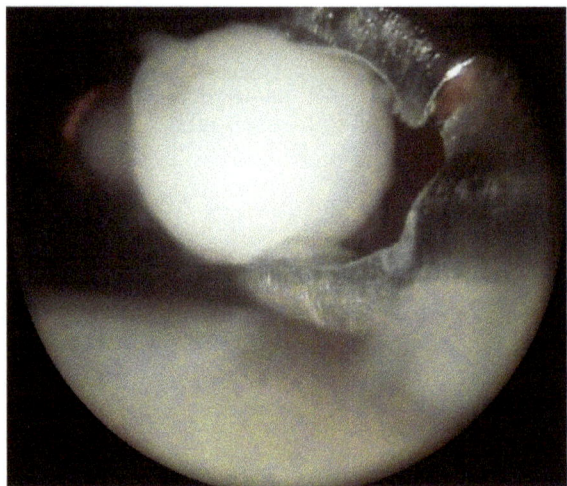

Fig. 14: Urology stone grasper with 3 prongs.

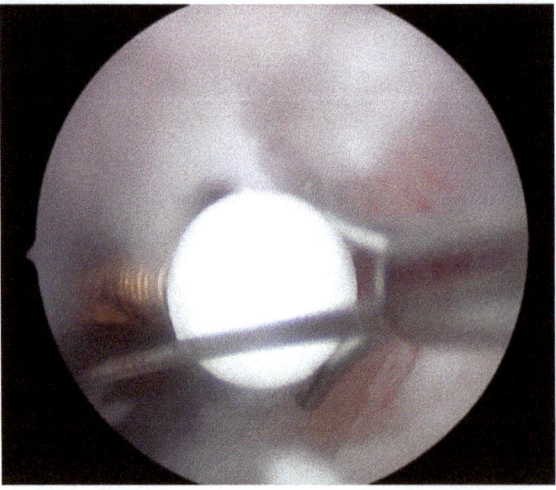

Fig. 13: CuT held with hysteroscopic grasper.

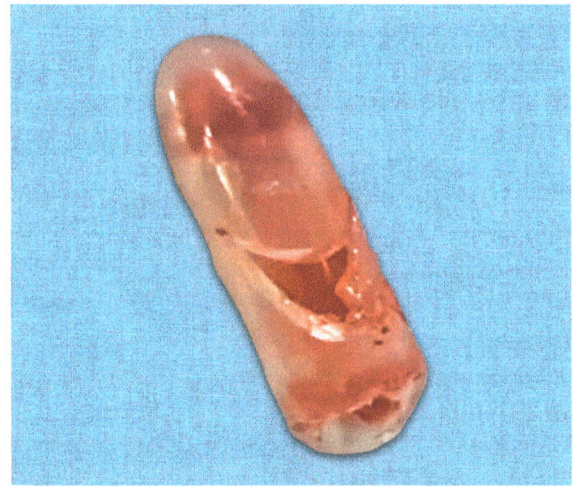

Fig. 15: Retrieved broken tip of Karman's cannula.

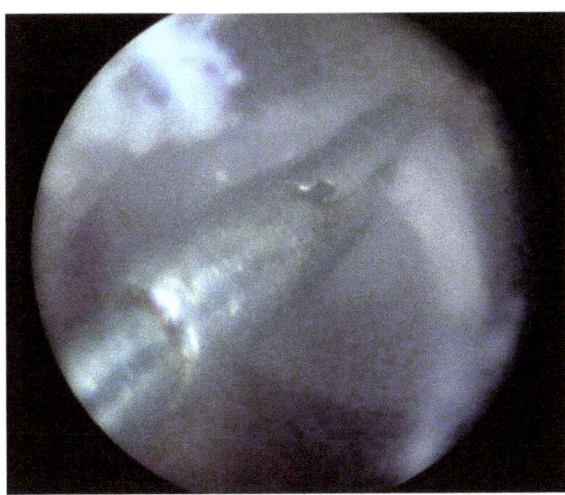

Fig. 16: Broken tip of the metal cannula during D and C.

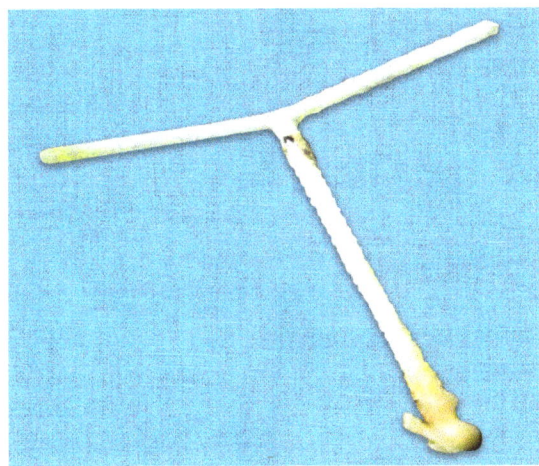

Fig. 17: CuT removed after 10 years of menopause.

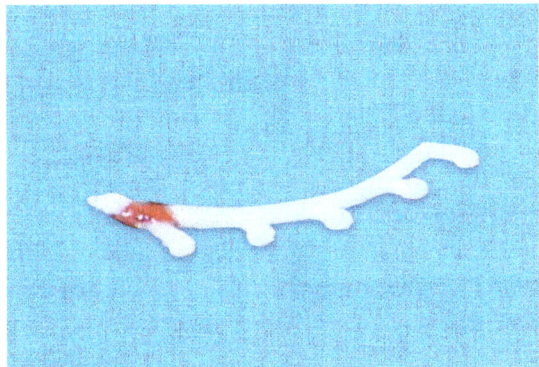

Fig. 18: Broken arm of multiload CuT after removal.

- *Laparoscopic intervention:* In rare cases where the foreign body cannot be accessed or removed hysteroscopically, laparoscopy may be required to remove it.

PREVENTION

To prevent the occurrence of misplaced foreign bodies in the uterine cavity, certain precautions can be taken:
- Proper insertion and regular check-ups of intrauterine devices to ensure they remain in the correct position.
- Awareness and caution during medical procedures involving the uterus to minimize the risk of leaving instruments behind.
- Educating individuals on proper hygiene practices and the correct use of tampons or other contraceptive devices.

CONCLUSION

Misplaced foreign bodies in the uterine cavity are an uncommon occurrence but can lead to significant health complications if left untreated. Early diagnosis and appropriate treatment can help to alleviate symptoms, prevent complications, and restore reproductive health. Retained intrauterine foreign bodies should be kept in mind for patients with recurrent vaginal discharge, unexplained chronic pelvic pain, and treatment-resistant abnormal uterine bleeding and infertility. In the era of minimal access surgery, hysteroscopy is the gold standard in management of misplaced foreign bodies in uterine cavity.

REFERENCES

1. Barsaul M, Sharma N, Sangwan K. 324 cases of misplaced IUCD—a 5-year study. Trop Doct. 2003;33(1):11-2.
2. Marchi NM, Castro S, Hidalgo MM, Hidalgo C, Monteiro-Dantas C, Villarroeal M, et al. Management of missing strings in users of intrauterine contraceptives. Contraception. 2012;86(4):354-8.
3. Lichtenberg ES. Complications of osmotic dilators. Obstet Gynecol Surv. 2004;59(7):528-36.
4. Camus M, Ropert JF, Iloki LH, Lefebvre G, Tranbaloc P. Endometrial ossification. Apropos of 5 recent cases. [Article in French]. J Gynecol Obstet Biol Reprod (Paris). 1990;19(3):295-300.
5. Umashankar T, Patted S, Handigund R. Endometrial osseous metaplasia: Clinicopathological study of a case and literature review. J Hum Reprod Sci. 2010;3:102-4.
6. CORONIS Collaborative Group, Abalos E, Addo V, Brocklehurst P, El Sheikh M, Farrell B, et al. Caesarean section surgical techniques: 3 year follow-up of the CORONIS fractional, factorial, unmasked, randomised controlled trial. Lancet. 2016;388:62-72.
7. Verma U, Astudillo-Davalos FE, Gerkowicz SA. Safe and cost-effective ultrasound guided removal of retained intrauterine device: our experience. Contraception. 2015; 12:52-3.

Chapter 15

Cervix Under Microscope

Luigi Montevecchi

■ INTRODUCTION

Every gynecologist knows perfectly what the cervix looks like, as it has been shown to him by his teachers, through the use of a vaginal speculum.

The luckiest ones also had the opportunity to learn the art of colposcopy, which allows you to observe—at macroscopic magnification up to a maximum of 20×—and distinguish the normal epithelium from the pathological one with the use of some reagents such as acetic acid and Lugol's solution.

But the great revolution took place thanks to Jacques Hamou's microcolpohysteroscope, which with the use of a vital dye (Waterman's blue ink) allows you to observe the lining cells of the uterine cervix in contact, up to a maximum of 150×.

■ NORMAL AND PATHOLOGICAL MICROSCOPIC ASPECTS OF THE UTERINE CERVIX

Before tackling a diagnosis with the microcolpohysteroscope, it is necessary to know the microscopic characteristics (normal and pathological) of the uterine cervix.

The tissue that covers the uterine cervix, which continues externally with the vaginal one, is made up of an epithelium, in which we can distinguish four layers: (1) Basal, (2) parabasal, (3) intermediate and (4) superficial **(Fig. 1)**: this is called squamous multilayered epithelium. The cells have a flat, polygonal appearance, and have a nucleus which progressively decreases in size from the deeper, more immature layers until it assumes a pyknotic appearance in the superficial cells. Therefore, a younger cell (= more immature) will assume a more rounded cytoplasm and its nucleus will occupy more space inside the cytoplasm, thus giving the impression—to

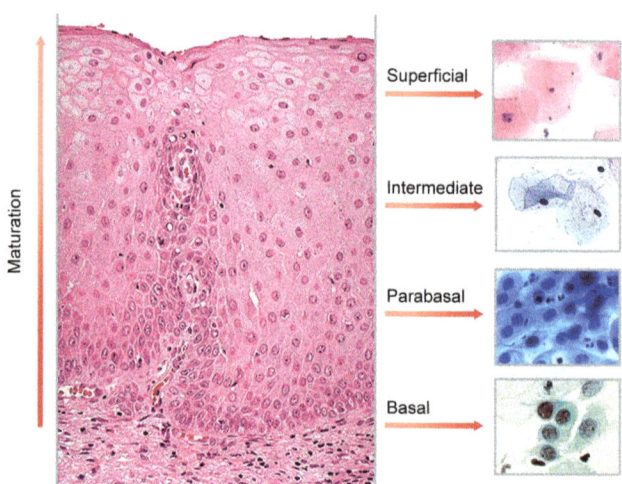

Fig. 1: Multilayered squamous epithelium of the uterine cervix.

a microscopic view of the tissue—of a greater nuclear "crowding" due to the scarcity of cytoplasm separating two contiguous cells.

On the contrary, the more mature surface epithelium—observed under the microscope, presents an appearance characterized by punctiform nuclei, widely spaced from each other, thanks to the greater amount of cytoplasm that separates them between two adjacent cells.[1]

The cervical canal is instead characterized by a single layer of elongated, cylindrical-shaped cellular elements which are arranged in papillary-type ridges and crypts which simulate the appearance of the glands: these cells are responsible for the production of mucus which we can observe macroscopically above all in the premenopausal patient during the ovulatory period. The junction line between the two epithelia (multilayered squamous and monostratified cylindrical) is defined as the squamo-cylindrical or squamocolumnar junction (SCJ) because of the elongated appearance of the cylindrical cells, similar

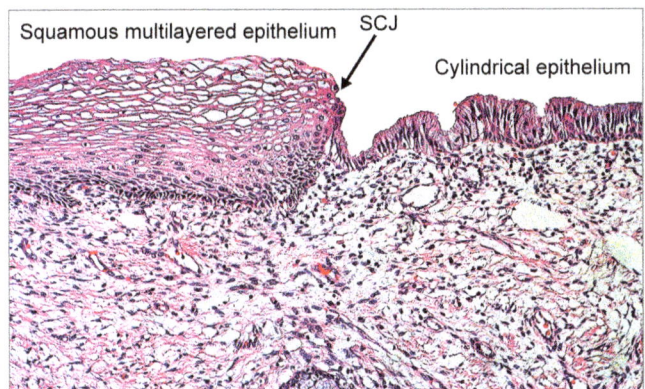

Fig. 2: The squamocolumnar junction (SCJ).

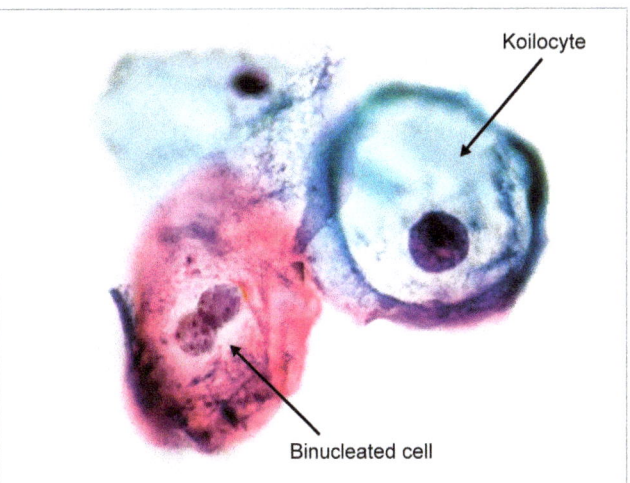

Fig. 3: Koilocyte and binucleated cell.

to columns **(Fig. 2)**. This area is particularly important—as all gynecologists know—as the site of the major cellular alterations, in the case of intraepithelial lesions of the uterine cervix. It is at this level, where there is a continuous rearrangement between the cylindrical epithelium and the squamous epithelium that the preneoplastic processes begin.

It should be remembered that there are other cells, which are frequently found on samples taken for cytology according to Papanicolaou (= pap smear): they are the elements of squamous metaplasia. This is a physiological phenomenon, which occurs regularly when the cylindrical cells, in contact with a traumatic, chemical, or inflammatory noxious agent (for example when they are in contact with the acidic vaginal environment), are replaced by pluripotent elements (stem or subcylindrical reserve cells) to form a more resistant multilayered epithelium.[2]

Squamous metaplasia cells have a morphology similar to basal or parabasal cells, a nucleus that occupies a large part of the cytoplasm, a rounded shape, and the characteristic of them all being the same size and regularly arranged when viewed by microcolpohysteroscope.

It is known that the main cause of the onset of cervical cancer and its precursors (low- or high-grade intraepithelial lesions) is the human papillomavirus (HPV). This, having come into contact with the multilayered epithelium of the uterine cervix, is able to penetrate inside the cells causing some characteristic modifications, which can be recognized under microscopic observation.

From the point of view of traditional cytology (that of the laboratory), there are three aspects that allow the diagnosis of viral infection to be made: koilocytosis, binucleation, and dyskeratosis. While the latter manifests itself only to the eye of the cytologist, after performing a traditional staining with the Papanicolaou technique, the other two alterations can also be easily observed with the microcolpohysteroscope, without the need to carry out any biopsy.

Koilocytosis (from the Greek κοῖλος = hollow) manifests itself with a perinuclear cytoplasmic halo, consisting of water only, does not contain glycogen and is negative for laboratory cytological staining with PAS (the PAS reaction—periodic acid–Schiff reagent—is a histochemical reaction, which highlights, by coloring them in magenta red, tissue components distinguished by glycolic groups).[3]

The nucleus appears enlarged, typical of the less mature layers, and the cytoplasm appears thickened at the periphery of the cell. Binucleated elements appear similar to koilocytes, except that they have two nuclei instead of one. Both elements thus manifest the cellular suffering due to the presence of the papillomavirus, preventing the maturation of the nucleus and the performance of some essential functions in the koilocytes, and in the binucleate cells the subdivision of the cytoplasm after the nuclear division, thus giving rise to a single cell with double nucleus **(Fig. 3)**.

MATERIALS AND METHODS

What is needed to perform a microcolpohysteroscopy?

This is—in a nutshell—the necessary material **(Fig. 4)**:
- Vaginal speculum
- Cotton
- Forceps

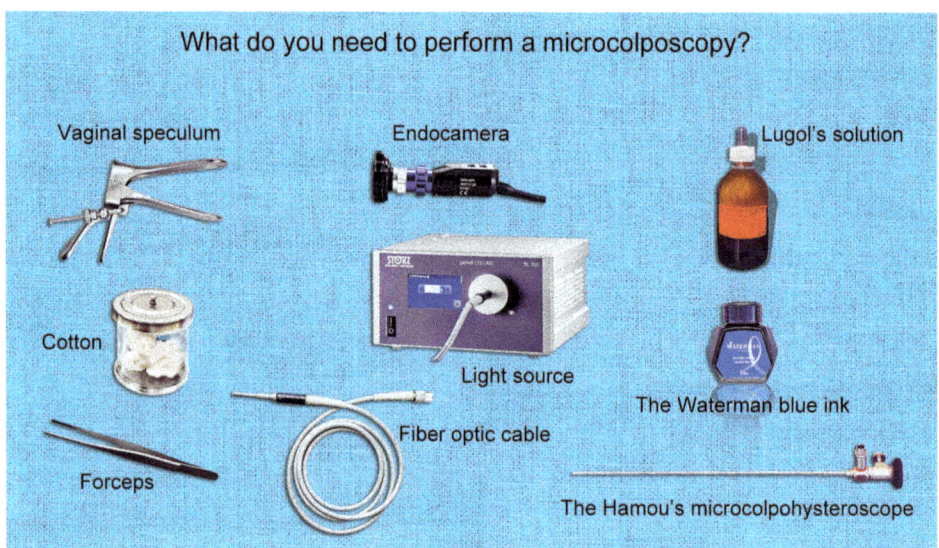

Fig. 4: Material needed for microcolpohysteroscopy.

- Light sources
- Fiber optic cable
- Video endoscopic camera
- Lugol's solution
- Hamou's microcolpohysteroscope
- Waterman's blue ink

It is absolutely important to remember that the Storz company of Tuttlingen (the only one to commercially produce Hamou's microcolpohysteroscope) made three models: the first (Hamou I) of 4.5 mm in diameter and characterized by a double eyepiece, was replaced toward the end of the 1980s by the second model (Hamou II), with maximum magnification up to 80×, and consisting of a single eyepiece. The latter, no longer on the market, was subsequently reduced in caliber (2.9 mm) and is not easy to find in all countries **(Fig. 5)**.

Weak Lugol's solution (4 grams of iodine, 8 grams of potassium iodide in 200 mL of purified water) can be purchased as it is prepared at the pharmacy, while Waterman's blue ink is a common ink for fountain pens and must be purchased at a stationery shop (or requested online) **(Fig. 6)**.

Vaginal speculum, cotton, forceps, light sources, fiber optic cable, and video endoscopic camera should be part of the equipment present in a hysteroscopist's office, and in any case, everyone can buy the system that best satisfies in terms of quality and price.

Once you have everything you need, how do you get optimal vision to be able to make a reliable diagnosis?

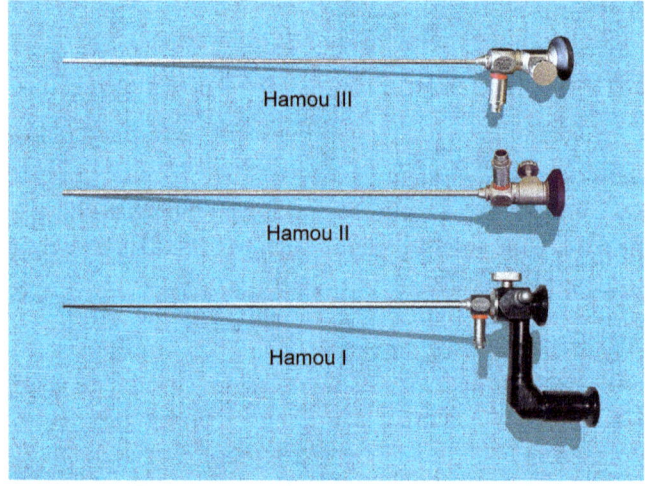

Fig. 5: Different types of Hamou's microcolpoisteroscope.

First, you will have to perform the normal bimanual exploration, to appreciate the possible presence of volumetric abnormalities and identify the mobility and position of the uterine cervix. Then you can insert the vaginal speculum in the right direction, so as to reduce the patient's discomfort. It may be sufficient to wet it with normal saline to reduce friction and facilitate insertion.

Once the uterine cervix has been correctly exposed, this—very probably—will be covered with mucus and/or secretions which reduce its view and hinder the correct application of the reagents in the subsequent phases: it is therefore necessary to carefully cleanse the

Cervix Under Microscope

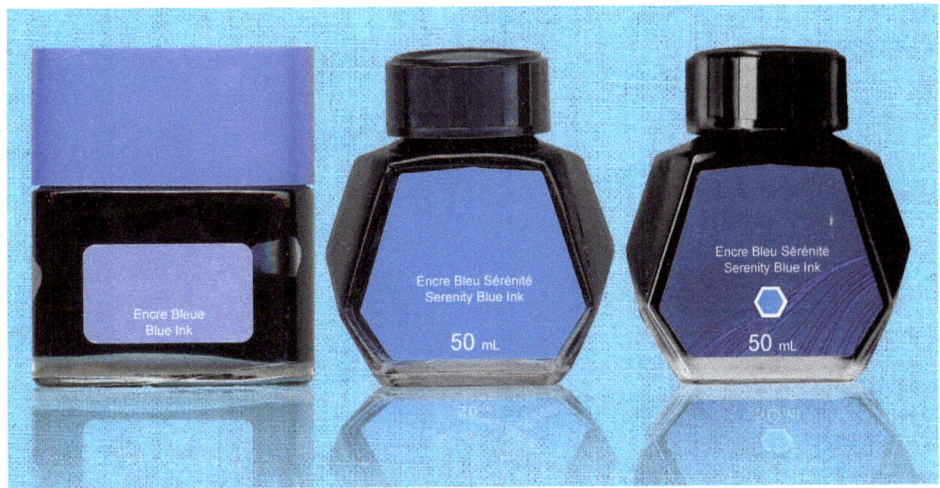

Fig. 6: Different bottles of Blue Waterman ink over the years.

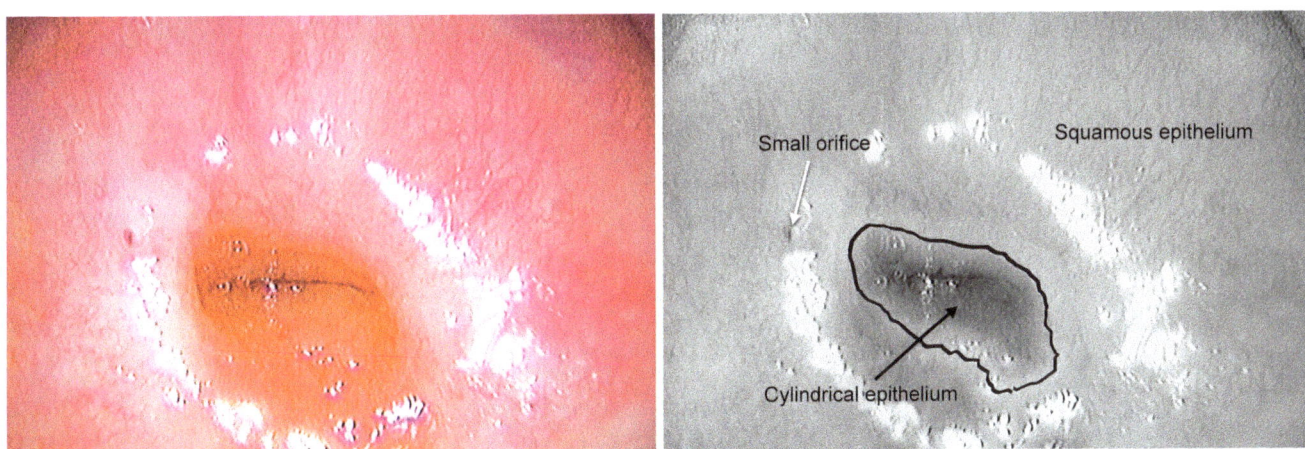

Fig. 7: Uterine cervix at 20× (microcolpohysteroscopy) without staining.

epithelium from the material which covers. This can be easily achieved using forceps and a saline-soaked cotton ball.

At this point, the observation of the uterine cervix at low magnification can begin, bringing the tip of the instrument close to about a couple of centimeters from the epithelium. In this way, a "macroscopic" view is obtained, similar to that of a traditional 10× colposcopy. We can distinguish the squamous epithelium, which surrounds the external uterine orifice, the cylindrical tissue, which immediately appears at the level of the cervical canal, and a small orifice, at 10 o'clock, probably made up of cylindrical epithelium **(Fig. 7)**.

The second stage of the microcolpohysteroscopic observation involves the application of Lugol's solution at the dilution already mentioned, so as to be able to highlight any immature areas (= not containing glycogen) which—consequently—do not take on the red-brownish color typical of mature squamous epithelium **(Fig. 8)**.

These areas will have to be subjected to a more careful microcolpohysteroscopic evaluation during the next phase: staining with Waterman's blue ink, and contact scanning for direct observation of the cervical cells without the need for sampling and sending to the laboratory.[2]

To observe the cells, Waterman's blue ink must be applied with a small cotton swab, both on the exocervical epithelium and within the first two centimeters of the cervical canal. After waiting about 10 seconds, the time required for it to be metabolized inside the cytoplasm and cell nucleus, remove the excess dye with a dry cotton ball. At this point, it is possible to bring the microcolpohysteroscope in contact with the epithelial surface, and operate the focus knob, to obtain an excellent view.

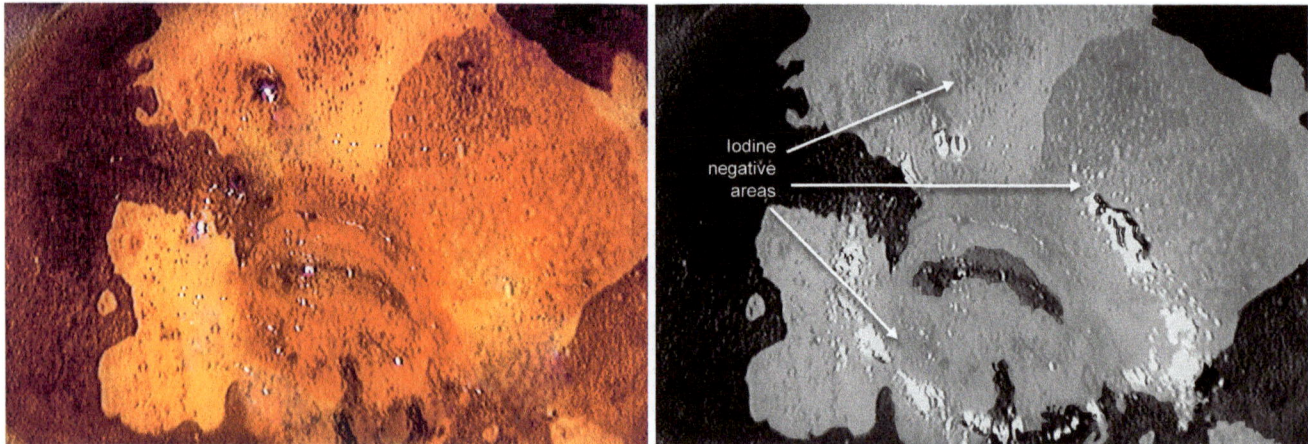

Fig. 8: Uterine cervix at 20× (microcolpohysteroscopy) after Lugol's solution.

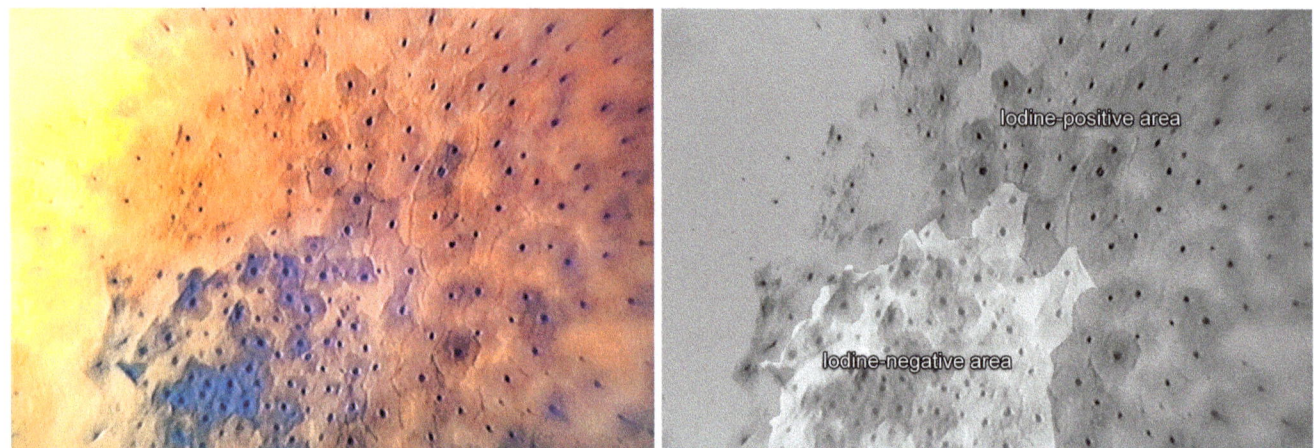

Fig. 9: Iodine-positive and iodine-negative areas (microcolpohysteroscopy 150×).

As can be seen from the images, the iodine-positive and iodine-negative epithelium, in this case, show a normal morphology (squamous cells, with a more or less mature nucleus, belonging to the superficial layers). It is thus possible to immediately exclude the presence of cellular abnormalities even on the areas which appeared not to take Lugol's solution **(Fig. 9)**.

The scan must proceed meticulously first on the anterior lip, then on the posterior one, along the SCJ. It should be remembered that the endocervical location of the junction, which makes traditional colposcopy unsatisfactory, does not substantially change the possibility of an adequate diagnosis in microcolpohysteroscopy: the characteristics of the instrument in fact allow us to observe this important marker with extreme precision even when it has ascended the cervical canal for many millimeters **(Fig. 10)**.

One of the major difficulties encountered by those who start practicing microcolpohysteroscopy is a clear vision. The main causes derive from the difficulty of keeping the end of the microcolpohysteroscope still in contact with the surface of the epithelium. It is essential to always have a foothold: to obtain it, you must hold the instrument as shown **(Fig. 11)**.

When the fiber optic cable is pointing downward and the focus knob is to the operator's left, the thumb and forefinger also "embrace" the axis of the instrument; conversely, if the cable is pointing upward, the knob of the microcolpohysteroscope is located to the right of the operator, and the fingers work more easily.

To avoid tremors, and consequently difficult if not impossible vision, remember to always maintain support on the rear branch of the speculum **(Fig. 12)**.

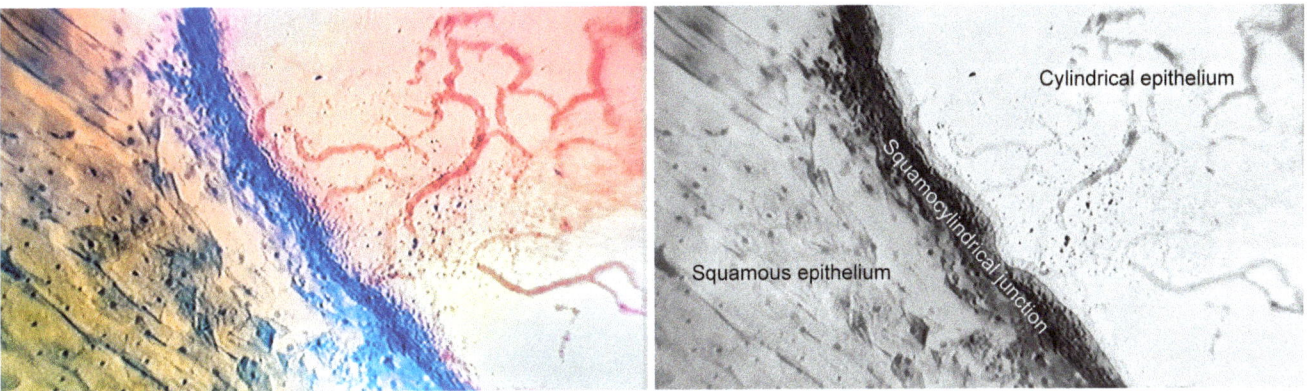

Fig. 10: The SCJ (microcolpohysteroscopy 150×). (SCJ: squamocolumnar junction)

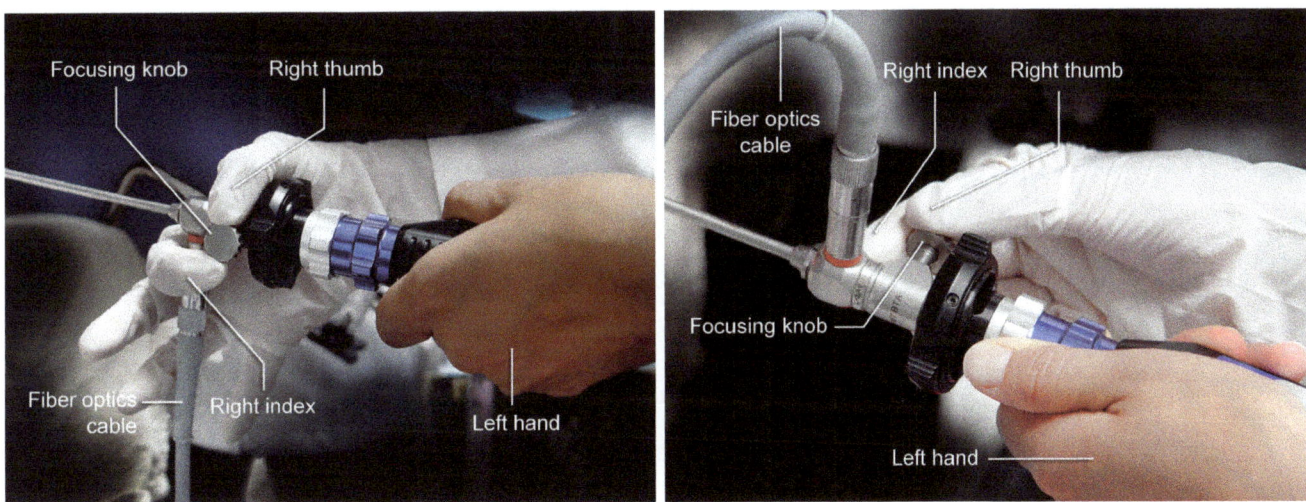

Fig. 11: How to hold the microcolpohysteroscope to focus.

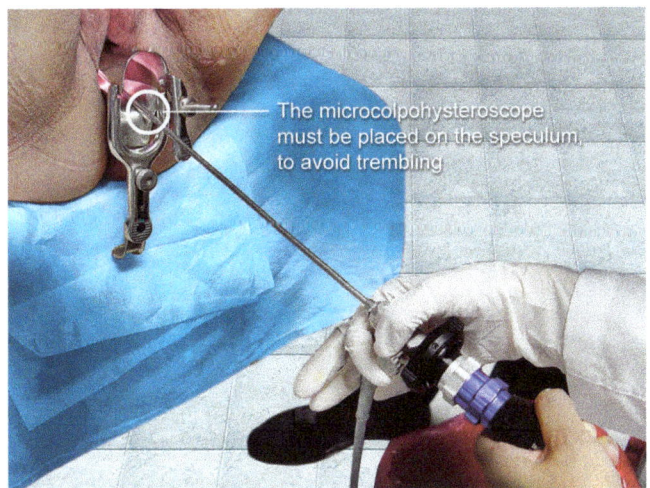

Fig. 12: How to hold the microcolpohysteroscope to prevent trembling.

When you have obtained a good dexterity, the cells of the uterine cervix will have no more secrets: you will immediately be able to distinguish between a normal epithelium and a pathological one; the appearance of the koilocytes and binucleated cells is practically superimposable on that previously illustrated in cytology, and the high-grade cellular alterations will be evident even to the eyes of the less expert (**Figs. 13 to 15**).[4]

CONCLUSION

Microcolpohysteroscopy is an easy-to-learn technique, which allows immediate outpatient diagnosis of preneoplastic lesions of the uterine cervix, without the need to carry out a biopsy sample and send it to the laboratory. Compared to traditional cytology (pap smear), it is able to establish the location and extent of any cellular alterations,

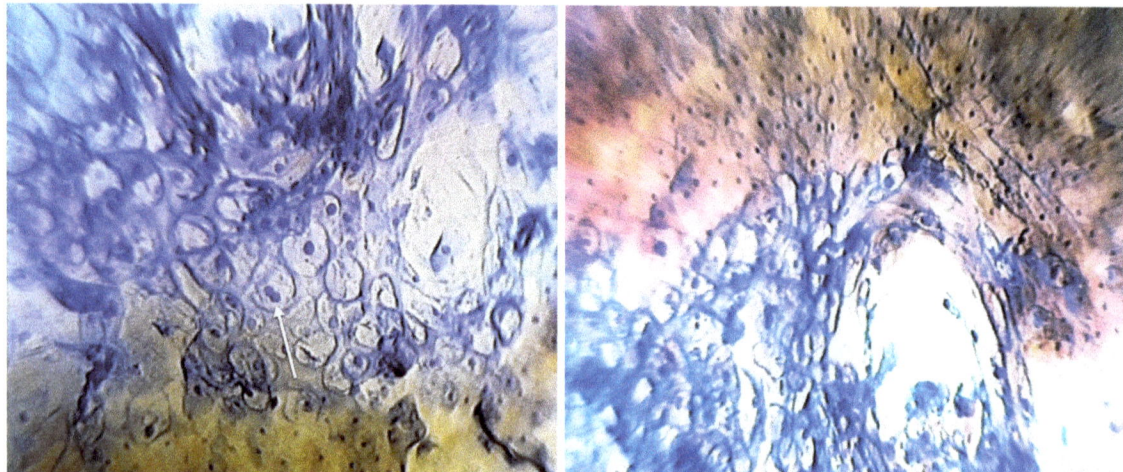

Fig. 13: Koilocytosis (microcolpohysteroscopy 150×).

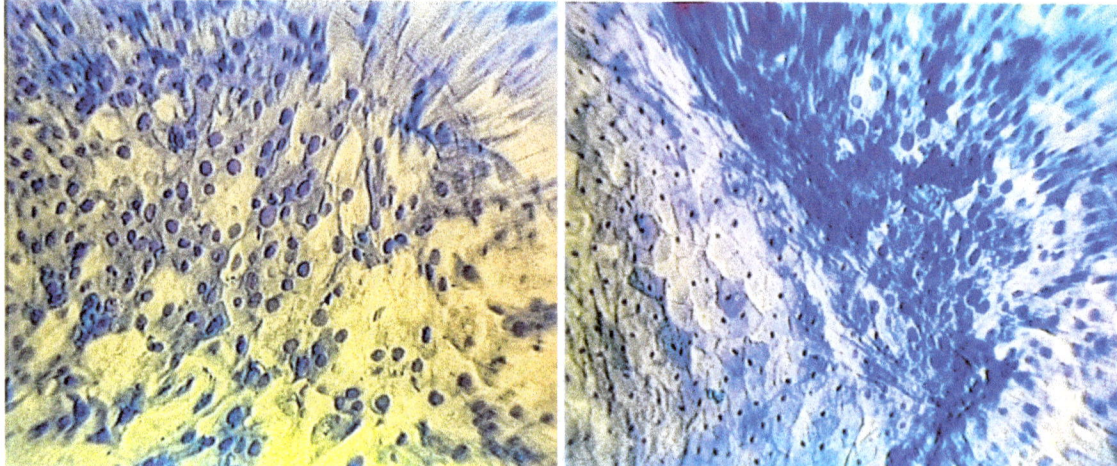

Fig. 14: High-grade squamous intraepithelial lesion (microcolpohysteroscopy 150×).

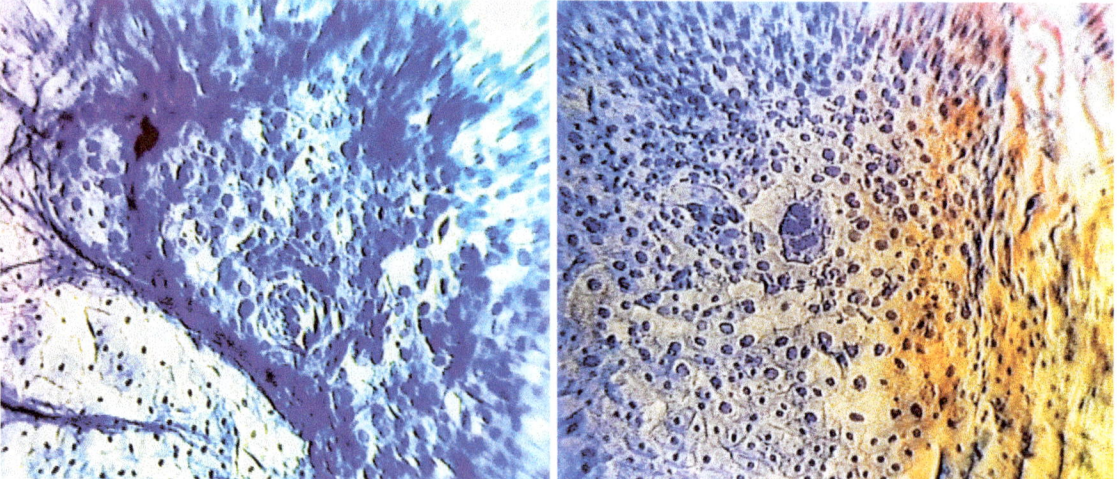

Fig. 15: High grade squamous intraepithelial lesion (microcolpohysteroscopy 150×).

compared to colposcopy it can observe the internal, endocervical border of the lesions and—consequently—know in advance the amount of tissue to be removed in case of excisional treatment.

REFERENCES

1. Hamou J. Microhistéroscopie: Une nouvelle technique en endoscopie et ses applications. Acta Endoscopica. 1980;10:415.
2. Montevecchi L, Vecchione A. (1986). Microcolpohysteroscopic features of cervical condylomatosis and their accuracy in detecting subclinical papillomavirus infection. [online] Available from: http://www.luigimontevecchi.it/files/Download/Microcolpohysteroscopic%20Features.pdf. [Last accessed November, 2023].
3. Montevecchi L. Microcolposcopia. In: Moscovitz T, Alonso L, Thcherniakovsky M (Eds). Tratado de Histeroscopia uma viagem pelas lentes do mundo. Di Livros Editora Ltda. 2021. pp. 125-48.
4. Montevecchi L, Drizi A. Diagnostic Hysteroscopy: vagina and cervix. Microcolpohysteroscopy—The Trocar. 2023; 4:34-44.

Hysteroscopy in Postmenopausal Bleeding

Chapter 16

Kalyan B Barmade, Pandit Palaskar, Manisha K Barmade

INTRODUCTION

Hysteroscopy is useful modality in the work up of patients with postmenopausal bleeding (PMB). The uterine cavity can be visualized directly and any abnormal areas identified precisely and the same taken for histopathological examination. Hysteroscopy is done nowadays by an office procedure which is valuable method for the patient and relatives. Hysteroscopy is gold standard for evaluation of cases with abnormal genital bleeding which includes PMB as well. It diagnoses the intrauterine lesions with precision. The lesions such as polyps, submucous fibroid, endometrial adenocarcinoma, and hyperplasia are diagnosed by hysteroscopy.[1]

A woman is considered menopausal, after cessation of menstruation for 1 year. The average age of menopause in Asian women is 46 years.[2]

General medical history, menstrual and obstetric history, duration since menopause, severity and duration of postmenopausal bleeding, history of gynecological operations, drug intake and associated symptoms.

A thorough general and systemic examination was done along with abdominal, vaginal, and rectal examination.

Clinical and sonographic evaluation followed by diagnostic and/or therapeutic hysteroscopy with office hysteroscope is to be done in all cases.

In each case, hysteroscopic visualization of the uterine cavity and hysteroscopic-guided biopsy needs to be done.

Atrophic endometritis (**Fig. 1**), endometrial hyperplasia (**Fig. 2**), and endometrial cancer are the leading causes of PMB.[3]

CAUSES OF POSTMENOPAUSAL UTERINE BLEEDING[4]

Causes of postmenopausal uterine bleeding are given in **Table 1**.

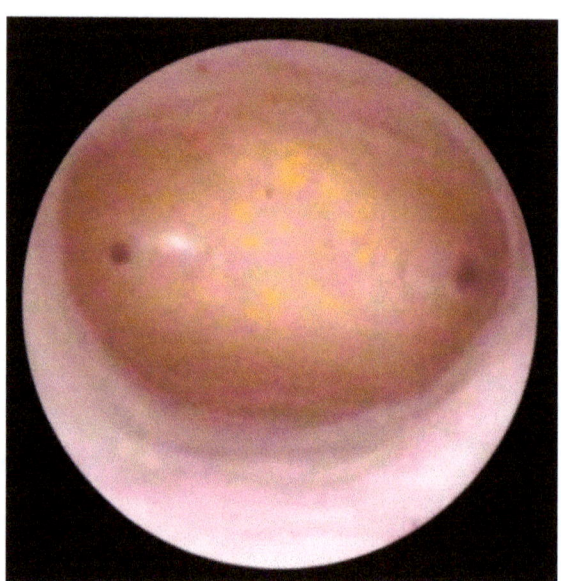

Fig. 1: Atrophic endometrium.

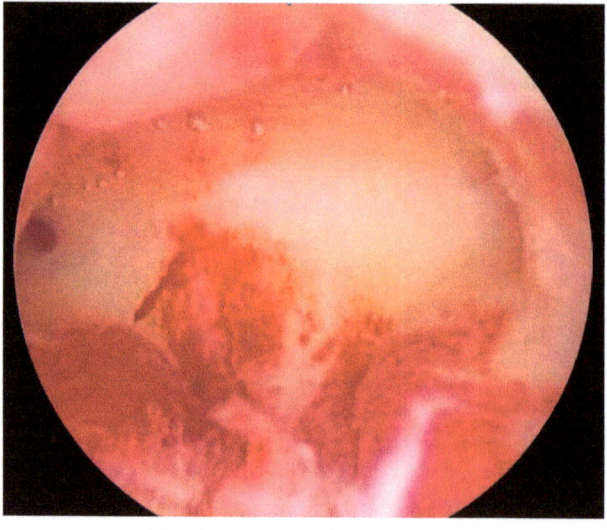

Fig. 2: Endometrial hyperplasia.

TABLE 1: Causes of postmenopausal uterine bleeding.[4]	
Causes of bleeding	**Percentage (%)**
Atrophic endometrium	60–80
Exogenous estrogens	15–25
Endometrial cancer	10
Endometrial polyps	2–12
Endometrial hyperplasia	5–10
Others (cervical cancer, urethral caruncle, trauma, etc.)	5–10

TABLE 2: Distribution of cases according to the age at menopause.[4]	
Age of attaining menopause (years)	**Number of women with PMB**
<45	3 (5)
45–49	8 (13.3)
50–55	34 (56.6)
>55	15 (25)
(PMB: postmenopausal bleeding)	

Around 60–70% of the patients with PMB had a thin endometrium (<5 mm) indicating atrophic endometrium as the most common cause.

Distribution of Cases According to the Age at Menopause[4]

Distribution of cases according to the age at menopause is given in **Table 2**.

CORRELATION BETWEEN ET ON TVS AND PMB[4]

Table 3 describes the correlation between endometrial thickness (ET) on transvaginal ultrasound (TVS) and PMB.

It is apparent that hysteroscopy is much more sensitive than TVS in the detection of focal endometrial pathology, and the specificity of hysteroscopy is more than TVS in diagnosing various endometrial conditions.

ON USG DIAGNOSIS

Diagnosis was made as follows:
- *Atrophic:* When the endometrium is homogenous and thin, endometrial thickness is ≤4 mm.

TABLE 3: Correlation between ET on TVS and PMB.[4]		
ET TVS (mm)	**Number of women with PMB**	**Percentage (%)**
<5	35	58.3
5–12	18	30
>12	7	11.6
(ET: endometrial thickness; PMB: postmenopausal bleeding; TVS: transvaginal ultrasound)		

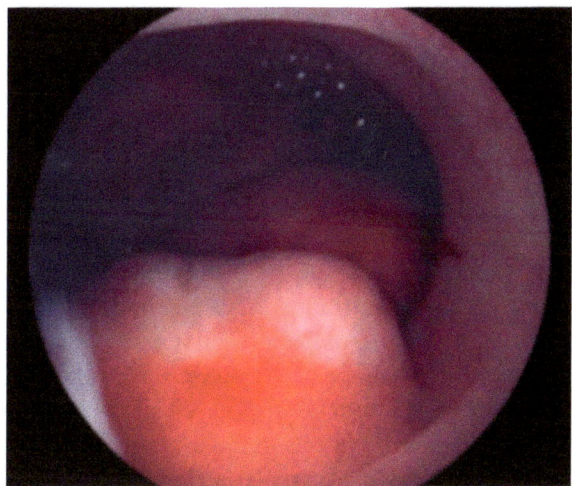

Fig. 3: Multiple polyps.

- *Thickened:* When the margins are regular with thickness 4 mm, endometrium is homogenous.
- *Polyp* **(Fig. 3)**: Focal endometrial thickening with regular margins
- *Hyperplasia:* Uniform diffuse thickening with thickness >10 mm
- *Carcinoma* **(Fig. 4)**: Thick heterogenous endometrium, irregular myoendometrial junction with absence of subendometrial halo.

HYSTEROSCOPY DIAGNOSIS

Under short general anesthesia, OR office hysteroscopy, hysteroscopy of 2.9 mm was introduced into the cervical canal under vision. Normal saline as the distension medium. The distension pressure inflated to 100 mm Hg, and maintained between 80 and 100 mm Hg. Endocervical canal, endometrial cavity and endometrial cavity inspection done in stepwise manner. Endometrial surface, color, vascularity, glandular pores, and tubal ostia were noted. Hysteroscopic biopsy taken and subjected for histopathology report. If there was suspicious areas, biopsy was taken from that area.

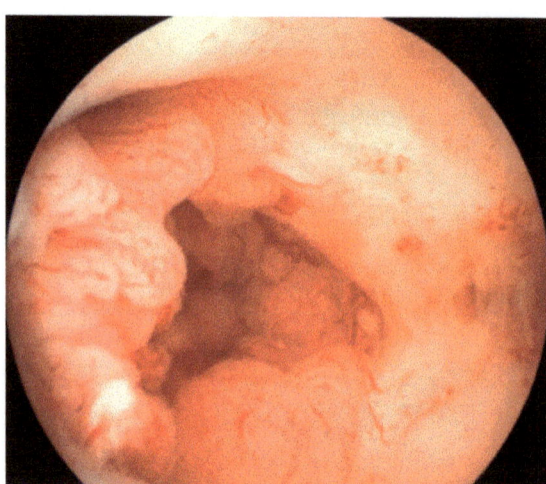

Fig. 4: Endometrial carcinoma.

Diagnosis by hysteroscopy was made on the following basis:
- *Atrophic:* Endometrium surface is pale, smooth, flat. Glandular opening and superficial vessels absent. Deep stromal vessels can be seen. Tubal ostia are obliterated.
- *Proliferative:* Endometrium surface looks smooth, pink relatively thick. Pores of endometrial glands seen with regularity. Superficial vascularization is relatively poor, tubal ostia are normal.
- *Secretory:* Smooth surface, velvety and red in appearance. Endometrium appears very thick. Superficial vessels appear in net-like geometrical pattern. Gland opening is seen, tubal ostia are seen.
- *Polyp:* Smooth surface, pink or white in color. Appears as uniform projection from the endometrium. Gland opening is seen. Vascularization is normal. Tubal ostia are visible.
- *Simple hyperplasia:* Rough surface, color is pink, yellow, or white. Height of the endometrium is very thick. Gland opening is seen. Rich superficial vascularization in network-like appearance is seen. Glandular orifice is seen. Tubal ostium is normal.
- *Complex hyperplasia:* Rough surface, color is pink, yellow, or white. Height of the endometrium is uneven and very thick. Rich superficial vascularization is seen with no specific pattern. Glandular orifice is seen but not well delineated. Tubal Ostium is normal.
- *Endometrial carcinoma:* Rough surface, papillary appearance with irregular polylobulated excrescence. Partially necrotic and hemorrhagic. Vascularization is irregular. Often clear demarcation can be seen between normal and cancerous endometrium.

CONCLUSION

Office hysteroscopy in women with PMB and an endometrium thickness of >4 mm offer the possibility of diagnosis as well as treatment in the same session.

A decision analysis regarding the diagnosis and treatment in women with PMB is necessary.

Hysteroscopy correlates more with histopathology when compared with transvaginal ultrasound. Hysteroscopy is superior and has higher efficacy in diagnosing endometrial abnormality in women with PMB.

REFERENCES

1. Torrejon R, Fernandez-Alba JJ, Carnicer I, Martin A. The value of hysteroscopic exploration for abnormal uterine bleeding. J Am Assoc Gynecol Laparosc. 1997;4(4):453-6.
2. Kaiser Daily Health Policy Report; January. 2007 Key findings from the Kaiser Women's Health Survey.
3. Pacheco JC, Kempers RD. Etiology of postmenopausal bleeding. Obstet Gynecol. 1968;32:40-6.
4. Tandulwadkar S, Deshmukh P, Lodha P, Agarwal B. Hysteroscopy in postmenopausal bleeding. J Gynecol Endosc Surg. 2009;1(2):89-93.

Expanded Scope of Hysteroscopy: Embryoscopy, Cesarean Section Scar Ectopic Pregnancy, Tubal Sterilization

Carugno Jose, Maria Chiara De Angelis, Sergio Haimovich

INTRODUCTION

Hysteroscopy has gained an important role in modern gynecology. It is considered the gold standard procedure for the evaluation and management of intrauterine pathology. In most cases, the intrauterine pathology can be diagnosed and treated in the same setting in the office applying the concept of "see and treat approach". Currently, more and more hysteroscopic procedures can be performed in the office setting. This is due to the feasibility of operative hysteroscopy using normal saline solution as a distending medium, the vaginoscopic approach, and the miniaturization of the instruments. Advances in technology have led to the miniaturization of high-definition hysteroscopes without compromising optical performance, thereby making hysteroscopy a simple, safe, and well-tolerated in the office setting.[1]

The modern development of hysteroscopy completely transformed the approach to uterine intracavitary pathologies, moving from a blind procedure under general anesthesia to an outpatient procedure performed under direct visualization. With the progress of technology, new indications have emerged. In this chapter, we will review innovative indications of hysteroscopic procedures in modern gynecology. Tips and tricks will be provided.

EXPANDED SCOPE OF HYSTEROSCOPY IN VAGINAL PATHOLOGY

The massive adoption of hysteroscopy in modern gynecology has revolutionized patient care. Conventional hysteroscopy involves introducing a speculum in the vagina and holding the cervix with a tenaculum to facilitate introducing the hysteroscope into the uterine cavity, but with the introduction of the "no-touch hysteroscopy" or "vaginoscopy" technique, there is no need for insertion of a speculum or the use of the tenaculum, making the procedure painless and better tolerated by patients.[2]

The vaginoscopic approach is useful in the evaluation of the vaginal canal and the cervix in cases of foreign bodies in the vagina in children, endometriosis of the rectovaginal septum in patients with dyspareunia,[3] mesh erosion as a complication of urinary incontinence, and/or pelvic organ prolapse surgery, infections, and other gynecologic conditions such as Müllerian anomalies, vaginal septum, double cervix among many others. Distension of the vaginal canal by fluid allows the direct visualization of the cervix and the vagina in a panoramic view **(Fig. 1)**.

Vaginoscopy is also advantageous in cases where preservation of the integrity of the hymen is desired. The diameter of the modern hysteroscopes ranges from 2.9 to 10 mm which can be easily inserted into the vagina through the hymen without causing any damage. Moreover, cases of vaginal endometriosis can be

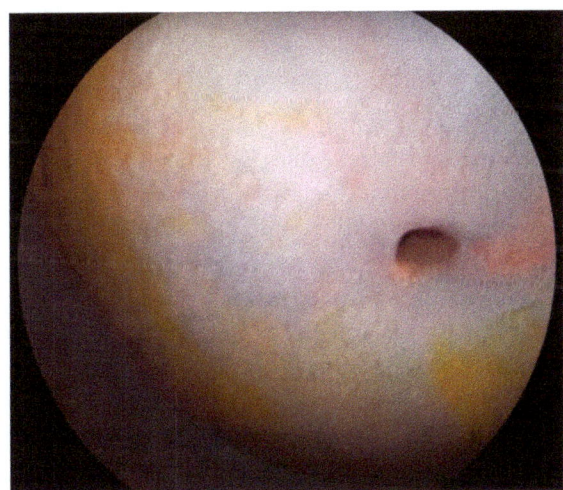

Fig. 1: Vaginoscopy offers direct visualization of the vagina and the cervix. In this image, appreciate the cervix and the external cervical os.

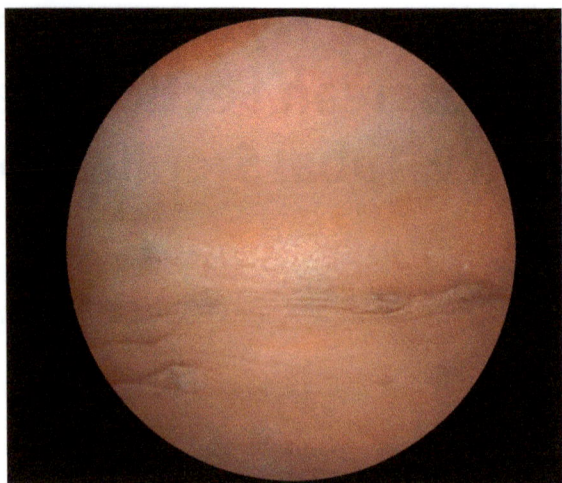

Fig. 2: Endometriosis of the rectovaginal septum.

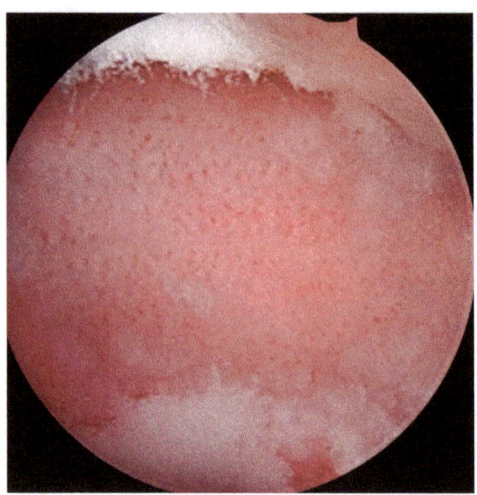

Fig. 4: Use of hysteroscopy in the evaluation of patients with vaginitis.

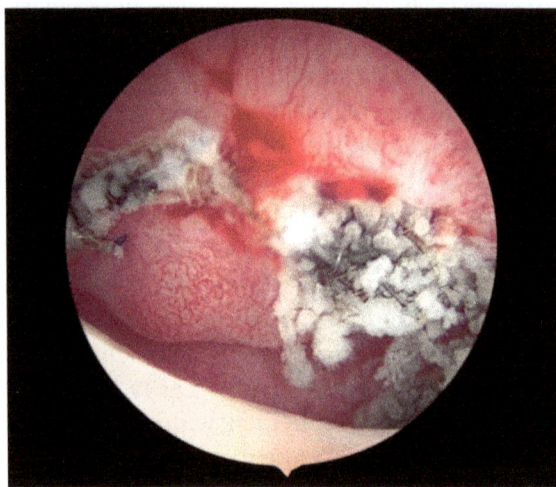

Fig. 3: Mesh erosion is identified and documented using vaginoscopy.

diagnosed vaginoscopically, through proper visualization and examination of the vagina **(Fig. 2)**. Bluish or brownish endometriotic spots which would have been missed by a conventional vaginal examination can now be seen. Rectovaginal deep infiltrating endometriosis is frequently implicated in cases of dyspareunia and can now be easily diagnosed and subsequently treated. Other conditions in which vaginoscopy plays a very important role are in the evaluation of mesh erosion after urinary incontinence or pelvic organ prolapse procedures in which mesh is placed. Mesh erosion can be easily visualized and documented using the hysteroscope **(Fig. 3)**. Also, some infectious conditions, such as yeast vaginitis, can be visually confirmed using vaginoscopy **(Fig. 4)**. The vaginoscopy technique is simple, easy to perform, and well tolerated by the patients. It is performed in four easy steps:

1. Introduction of the tip of the hysteroscope into the vagina
2. Obliteration of the vulva to allow the accumulation of fluid in the vaginal canal
3. Visualization of the posterior cul-de-sac and identification of the uterine external cervical os
4. Accessing the uterine cavity

In conclusion, vaginoscopy permits the visualization of the vagina and allows an atraumatic insertion of the hysteroscope into the uterine cavity.

Key Points

- Vaginoscopy is an innovative approach that allows the direct evaluation and image documentation of vaginal pathology.
- It allows the access of the uterine cavity protecting the integrity of the hymen when needed.
- It is a painless approach for the insertion of the hysteroscope into the uterine cavity.
- It is a simple technique that can be easily learned and adopted by the gynecologist with minimal effort.

EXPANDED SCOPE OF HYSTEROSCOPY IN THE EVALUATION OF THE CERVIX

The cervix is the lowermost portion of the uterus and provides both transport and protective function to the uterine cavity. The external cervical os, the endocervical canal, and the internal cervical os must be passed through to access

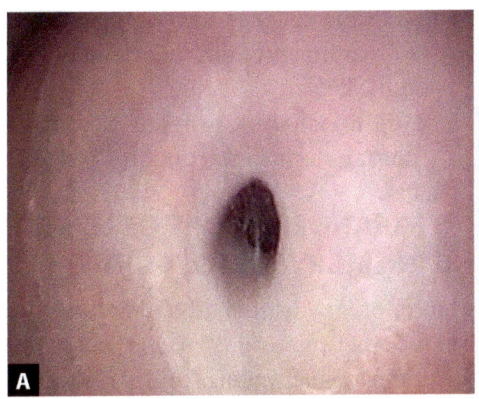 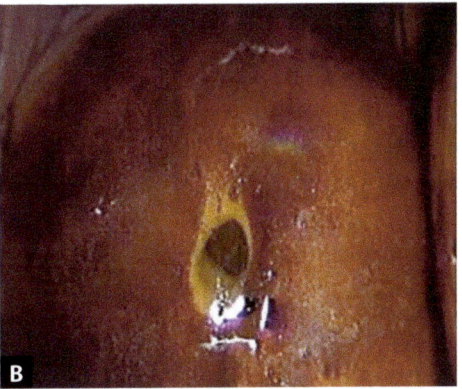

Figs. 5A and B: Normal uterine cervix before (A) and after (B) application of Lugol's solution.
Courtesy: Images by Professor L Montevecchi

the uterine cavity. Visualization of the cervical canal is an integral part of modern hysteroscopy. Different pathology is encountered at the level of the cervix. The visualization and recognition of the structures of the endocervical canal are important to avoid a common hysteroscopic complication such as the creation of a false passage.

Hysteroscopy allows the examination of the vagina, the ectocervix, as well as the cervical canal with clear direct visualization of the structures. Both the vaginal and ectocervical mucosa are covered by a stratified squamous epithelium and appear in a pale pinkish color when visualized with the hysteroscope. The cervix can display normal or abnormal features which are visible in hysteroscopy: mucus, ectropion, ectocervical polyps, cysts, adhesions, and endometriosis implants among other.

Microcolpohysteroscopy (MCH) is performed visualizing the uterine cervix by placing a speculum inside the vagina. Lugol's solution is then applied on the cervix. The areas that capture the Lugol's solution are those rich in glycogen. The color turns dark brown **(Figs. 5A and B)**.

After this initial superficial evaluation of the cervix, the tissue cervix is painted with Waterman's blue ink. The ink penetrates into the cytoplasm of the cells and the nucleus of the mature squamous epithelium, and into the cells undergoing squamous metaplasia, leaving the cylindrical epithelium colorless **(Fig. 6)**. This feature allows an easy differentiation between squamous and cylindrical epithelium, making it easy to identify the squamous–cylindrical junction, so important for the study of preneoplastic lesions of the uterine cervix.

Key Points

- The evaluation of the cervix is an important part of the gynecologic examination.

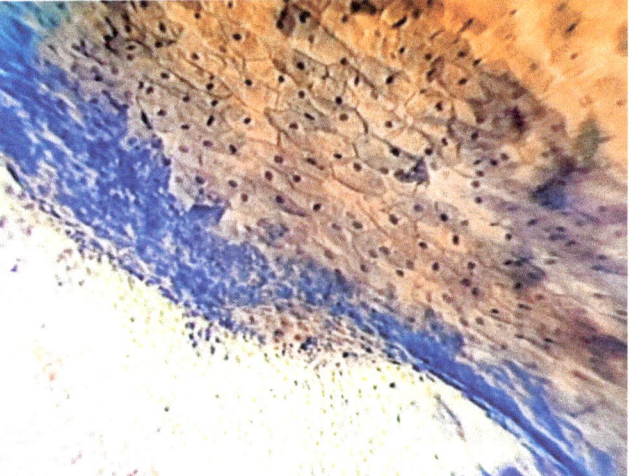

Fig. 6: The squamocolumnar junction (SCJ) (microcolpohysteroscopy 150×): Bottom left: unstained cylindrical epithelium; top right: mature superficial squamous epithelium; blue cells: transformation zone.
Courtesy: Image by Professor L Montevecchi

- The technique to evaluate the cervix is easy to adopt but requires training and expertise.
- Microcolpohysteroscopy allows the evaluation of cervical pathology and could represent an alternative to conventional colposcopy.

EXPANDED SCOPE OF HYSTEROSCOPY IN INTRAUTERINE STERILIZATION

Hysteroscopic intrauterine sterilization has always gained much attention in the gynecologic community. Three systems became available on the market: (1) in 1988 the Ovabloc Intra Tubal Device (Advanced Medical Grade Silicones BV), (2) in 2002 the Essure system (Conceptus Incorporated), and (3) in 2009 the Adiana Permanent

Contraception system (Hologic, Inc.) **(Figs. 7A and B)**. The Ovabloc device is a silicon mixture that is instilled into the tubal ostium and solidifies within 5 minutes into a rubber plug which occludes the tubal lumen providing permanent sterilization. The Essure device is a 4 cm expanding spring made of a nitinol outer coil and stainless-steel inner coil with polyethylene terephthalate fibers that is placed in the proximal section of the fallopian tube using the hysteroscope. The Adiana sterilization technique is a combination of 60 seconds of radiofrequency appliqued to the mucosa of the fallopian tube followed by deployment of a 3.5 mm matrix into the created lesion. These distinct mechanisms of action may lead to differences in feasibility and effectiveness of the different intrauterine sterilization modalities.[4]

Considering feasibility, the 78–98% probability of successful placement at first attempt, and the 90–100% verified by a proper confirmation test, all three hysteroscopic sterilization techniques have sufficient success rates. Adiana and Essure have the highest successful placement rates, 94% and range, 81–98%, respectively, versus Ovabloc, range, 78–84%.

Although initially successful and effective, unfortunately, all three devices were taken off the market after a short period of clinical use. Ovabloc was removed from the market in 2009 because of high failure rates and difficulty with maintaining cold storage with silicone. The Adiana device was removed from the market in 2012 because of its high failure rates and inability to keep up with legal costs over patent infringement litigation. The Essure device was voluntarily removed from the market by Bayer in December 2018 due to multiple law suits filed against the device.[5]

Key Points

- Hysteroscopic sterilization is a great minimally invasive sterilization option.
- Multiple devices have appeared on the market but were removed from the market after a brief period of clinical use.
- Additional work is needed to create the ideal intrauterine sterilization option.

EXPANDED SCOPE OF HYSTEROSCOPY IN EMBRYOFETOSCOPY

Embryoscopy is defined as the direct visualization of the embryo between 5 and 8 weeks' gestational age. Fetoscopy is the direct visualization of the fetus after 8 weeks of gestation.[6]

Recent evolution in fiberoptic technology has led to miniaturization of endoscopic equipment allowing to perform the procedure during the 1st trimester, thus giving it a new perspective.

Embryofetoscopy represents an exciting technique for visualizing the 1st-trimester embryo and fetus **(Figs. 8 to 10)**. Evolution in hysteroscopic instruments and changing trends toward 1st trimester prenatal diagnosis have given new potentials to this "old" technique. Embryoscopy can

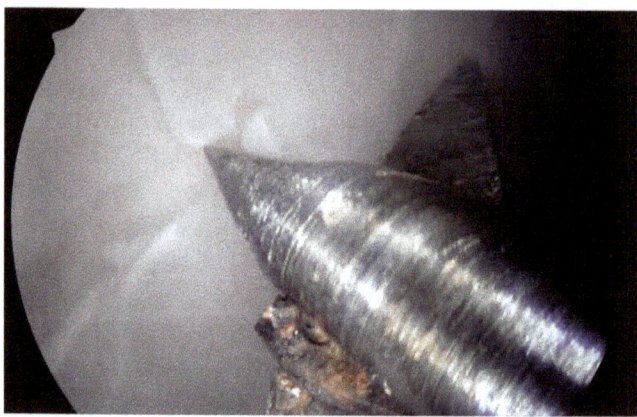

Fig. 8: Opening of the gestational sac using hysteroscopic scissors.

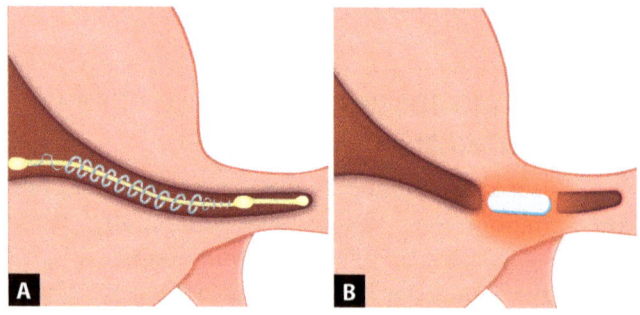

Figs. 7A and B: (A) The coil of the Essure device in place; (B) The Adiana matrix.

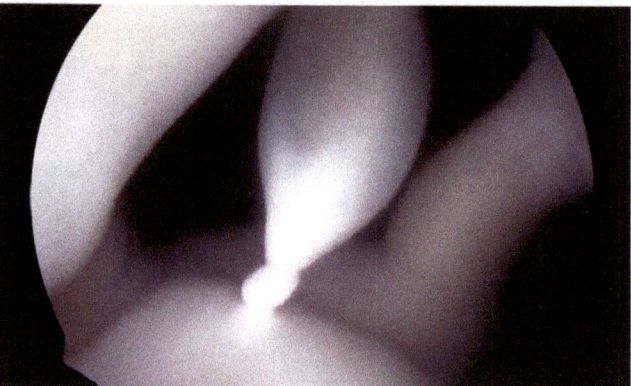

Fig. 9: Umbilical cord stricture.

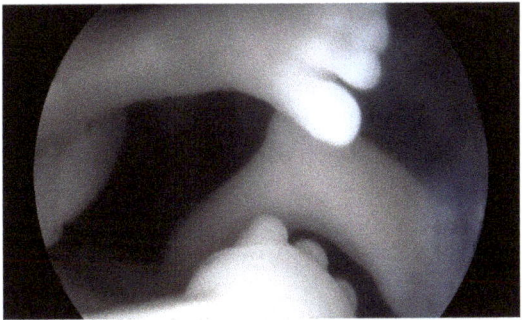

Fig. 10: Detailed visualization of the fetal parts is identified.

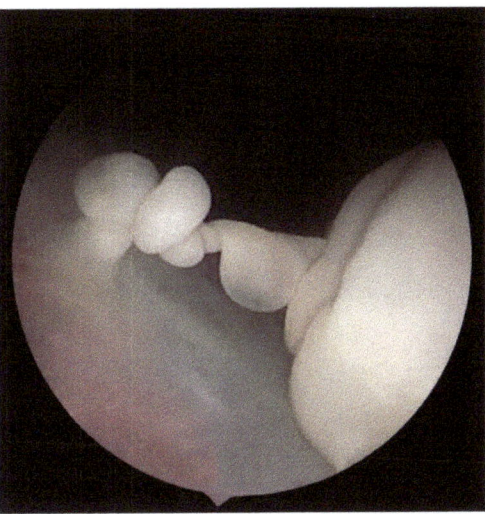

Fig. 12: Visualization of the umbilical cord revealing abnormal coiling with clear stricture of the cord.
Courtesy: Image by Professor Sergio Haimovich

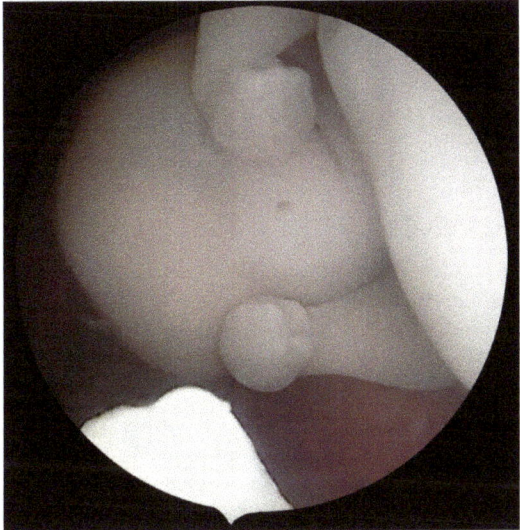

Fig. 11: Embryonic view revealing malformation of both hands.
Courtesy: Image by Professor Sergio Haimovich.

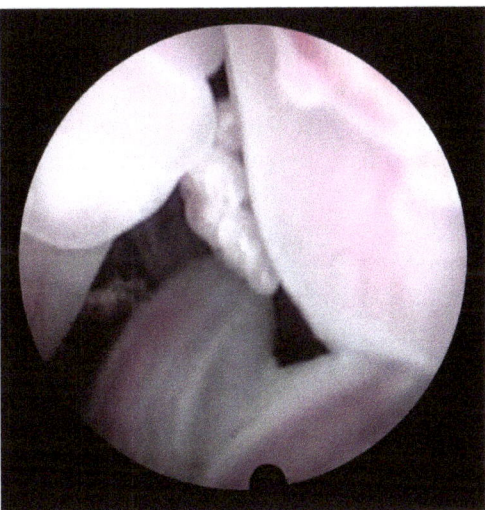

Fig. 13: Embryofetal parts visualized inside the ectopic gestational sac.

be applied in women desiring to terminate the pregnancy and can prove an indispensable tool for confirming and clarifying our knowledge of embryonic development, since key embryo structures and developmental milestones can be visualized closely. Embryofetoscopy can additionally permit access to the embryonic circulatory system for early fetal blood sampling. Embryofetoscopy in missed abortions is free of this risk and provides us with information on the causes responsible for the failed embryonic developmental steps so that parents can be effectively counseled about future pregnancies **(Figs. 11 and 12)**.

Key Points

- Embryofetoscopy is gaining an important role in prenatal diagnosis.
- It is a new promising technique that requires further development.
- Clinical indications of embryofetoscopy are expanding.

EXPANDED SCOPE OF HYSTEROSCOPY IN ECTOPIC PREGNANCY

Hysteroscopic removal of ectopic pregnancy is the latest option in the management of cervical ectopic pregnancy where the products of conception can be identified within an enlarged area of the cervical canal, the product of conception can be removed using bipolar resectoscope, and the blood vessels can be ablated simultaneously **(Figs. 13 and 14)**. Complete resection through hysteroscopy under direct visualization helps in preventing hemorrhage, promotes resolution, and

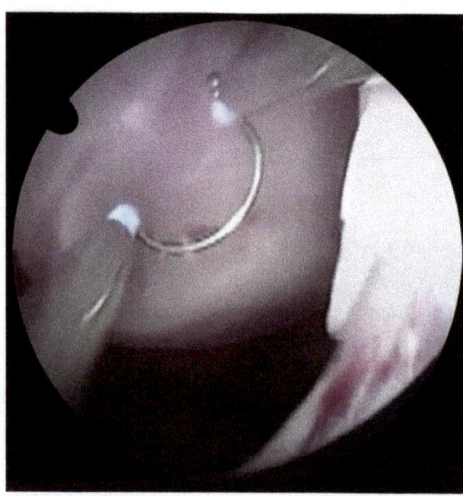

Fig. 14: Use of the bipolar hysteroscopic resectoscope for the extraction of the ectopic pregnancy and coagulation of the vessels if needed.

avoids prolonged follow-up in cases of cervical ectopic pregnancy. The visualization of normal uterine cavity with the entire gestational sac embedded in the wall below the internal os is considered a definitive diagnosis.

Cervical ectopic pregnancies are difficult to treat. Early diagnosis and medical management with systematic or local administration of methotrexate are the treatments of choice. Conservative approaches in late stages have proven beneficial in preserving a women's fertility. Hysteroscopic resection is a potentially safe and effective option for fertility-sparing management of patients with cervical ectopic pregnancy.

Key Points

- The diagnosis and management of cervical ectopic pregnancy represent a challenge for the clinician.
- The hysteroscope could play an important role in the management of nontubal ectopic pregnancies.
- Further clinical experience is needed before recommending the routine use of hysteroscopy in the management of ectopic pregnancy.

CONCLUSION

Hysteroscopy is gaining a very important role in modern gynecology. With the development of new miniaturized instruments with great improvement of the quality of the scope, the indications for hysteroscopic procedures are always increasing. New indications and new procedures are frequently described. Appropriate training is mandatory when incorporating new hysteroscopic diagnostic and therapeutic hysteroscopic procedures into clinical practice.

REFERENCES

1. Salazar CA, Isaacson KB. Office Operative Hysteroscopy: An Update. J Minim Invasive Gynecol. 2018;25(2):199-208.
2. Bettocchi S, Selvaggi L. A vaginoscopic approach to reduce the pain of office hysteroscopy. J Am Assoc Gynecol Laparosc. 1997;4(2):255-8.
3. Di Spiezio Sardo A, Di Iorio P, Guida M, Pellicano M, Bettocchi S, Nappi C. Vaginoscopy to identify vaginal endometriosis. J Minim Invasive Gynecol. 2009;16(2):128-9.
4. la Chapelle CF, Veersema S, Brolmann HA, Jansen FW. Effectiveness and feasibility of hysteroscopic sterilization techniques: a systematic review and meta-analysis. Fertil Steril. 2015;103(6):1516-25.e1-3.
5. Murthy P, Edwards J, Pathak M. Update on hysteroscopic sterilisation. Obstet Gynaecol. 2017;19(3):227-35.
6. Paschopoulos M, Meridis EN, Tanos V, O'Donovan PJ, Paraskevaidis E. Embryofetoscopy: a new "old" tool. Gynecol Surg. 2006;3(2):79-83.

Chapter 18

Anticipating, Preventing, and Managing Complications in Hysteroscopy

Patrícia Nazaré, José Luís Metello

INTRODUCTION

Hysteroscopy is a minimally invasive, safe, and well-tolerated technique, with a low complication rate. Complications are more common in surgical versus diagnostic hysteroscopy (0.95% vs. 0.13%).[1] Adhesiolysis and myomectomy are the procedures with more complications (up to 4.5%). Although rare, some can be life-threatening, so it is important to know how to avoid or identify them. Intraoperative complications include:
- False pathways, uterine perforation (0.12–3%)
- Cervical laceration (0.9%)
- Hemorrhage (0.03–0.61%)
- Infection (0.01–1.42%)
- Visceral-bladder or bowel lesion (0.02%)
- Fluid intravasation/overload (0.20%)
- Gas embolism (0.03–0.09%)
- Electrosurgical injury, vasovagal reaction, and intrauterine adhesions
- Anesthetic complications.[1,2]

COMPLICATIONS RELATED TO PATIENT

Positioning of Patient

The patient is placed in the dorsal lithotomy position. Correct positioning is essential, otherwise there may be injury to the femoral, peroneal, or sciatic nerve. Flexion, abduction, and external rotation of the thigh should be minimized. To prevent injury to the peroneal nerve, the leg should be placed on a padded surface, to avoid compression against a hard surface.[3,5]

Comorbidities

The appropriate patient selection for this procedure is based not only on the size and depth of the lesion, availability of appropriate materials, and the operator's experience, but also on the patient's predisposition considering other comorbidities such as diabetes, hypertension, obesity, cardiac function, previous uterine surgery, cervical disease, and vaginal atrophy.[2]

COMPLICATIONS RELATED TO INSTRUMENT AND METHODS

Cervical Dilation

About half of the complications of hysteroscopy happen during the cervical canal passage. According to the diameter of the hysteroscope used, sometimes prior cervical dilation may be required.

There is not enough evidence to recommend routine cervical ripening and individual risk factors (including postmenopausal status, nulliparity, previous cervical trauma, or other cervical procedures) should be evaluated.[2] Cervical dilation can be done preoperatively with prostaglandins (200 or 400 μg vaginal or oral, at least 2–4 hours before the procedure) or osmotic dilators. Osmotic dilators require insertion the day before, which is why they are not routinely applied. The dilation can also be mechanical, which is usually done during the procedure. Adjunctive treatment with vaginal estrogen may be combined (daily for 2 weeks prior to the procedure).

Intraoperatively, this difficulty can be overcome using a hysteroscope with hydrodissection under direct visualization. If there is scar tissue, it can be debrided with scissors or tweezers. Simultaneous ultrasound can help to guide the instruments through the correct path. The blind insertion of small instruments should be avoided as they can create false paths and lead to uterine perforation.[1]

Resectoscope and Electric Current

During the use of electric current, electrosurgical injury to adjacent organs (bowel, bladder, and pelvic vessels) may occur due to its thermal effects. This risk is particularly high during septotomy, deep infiltration fibroids, or when using coagulation near tubal ostia. To prevent thermal injury, the energy source should not be activated without a clear visualization of uterine cavity and must be moving whenever it is activated, thus the temperature does not increase too much at a specific point.

Distension Media: Gas Embolism and Fluid Overload

Fluid

Fluid distension is achieved with isotonic fluid (saline solution or ringer's lactate) or hypotonic fluid (sorbitol, mannitol, or glycine). The isotonic distension media is currently the most widely used. The main risk of these means of distension is fluid overload, by excessive fluid absorption, which can be expected when there is a fluid deficit of >1,000 cc with hypotonic solution or 2,500 cc with isotonic solution. Fluid deficit is affected by the number and size of excised lesions, depth of resection, intrauterine pressure, duration of the procedure, and the patient's blood pressure and comorbidities.[2] To prevent complications, the procedure should be stopped when a fluid deficit of 2,500 cc or 1,000 cc for isotonic or hypotonic fluid is reached, respectively (in patients with comorbidities, 1,500 cc or 750 cc, respectively). To cross the cervical canal, higher fluid pressures (100–120 mm Hg) are usually required, and within the cavity, the pressure should be decreased to a minimum value that allows adequate visualization (50–80 mm Hg).[1]

Signs of fluid overload include nausea, headache, dyspnea, chest pain, visual disturbances, and agitation. Without treatment, it can progress to seizures, pulmonary edema, and cardiorespiratory arrest.[5] If volume overload is suspected, pulmonary auscultation, vital monitoring, chest X-ray (if pulmonary edema is suspected), and measurement of serum electrolyte levels should be considered. Treatment consists of limiting the entry of fluids, increasing diuresis (furosemide 20–40 mg IV) and correcting hyponatremia. If sodium values <125 mEq/L, intensive care support should be sought. Symptoms such as acute neurological changes or nausea/vomiting constitute a medical emergency.

Gas

Gas distension uses CO_2. Currently, the use of gas as distension media is rare. Gas embolism with CO_2 is rare because it is very soluble in plasma. However, ambient air is poorly soluble, and its embolization can lead to cardiovascular collapse. To avoid gas embolism, the most serious complication of surgical hysteroscopy, the Trendelenburg position should be avoided, CO_2 flow should be <100 cc/min, intrauterine pressure should be between 70 and 100 mm Hg (and lower than mean arterial pressure), air bubbles should be purged before hysteroscope introduction, avoid deep myometrial resections, minimize cervical trauma, and limit multiple reinsertions of the hysteroscope into the uterine cavity.[1]

The signs/symptoms of gas embolism are dyspnea, chest pain, hypotension, tachycardia, decreased expired CO_2, oxygen desaturation, and mill wheel murmur. The procedure should be stopped immediately, and the emergency resuscitation team should be called. Some maneuvers that can be done immediately are the placement of the patient in the left lateral decubitus position (Durant's maneuver), emptying the uterus and occluding the vagina with wet gauze to prevent the entry of air through the cervix.[3,4]

■ COMPLICATIONS RELATED TO PATHOLOGY

Many of the complications of hysteroscopy stem from difficulty in entering the uterine cavity through the cervical canal and manipulation of instruments, namely the creation of false pathways, uterine perforation, cervical lacerations, vasovagal reactions, and significant hemorrhage.

Uterine Perforation

This complication is the most frequent and usually occurs at the beginning of the procedure, before establishing a clear path to the uterus. Risk factors are cervical stenosis, blind insertion of instruments, postmenopausal period, previous cervical/intrauterine procedures or anatomical distortion (extreme anteversion or retroversion, congenital anomalies, and intrauterine adhesions).[2] To avoid this complication, a complete medical history and physical examination (namely size and position of the uterus) should be done to identify the risk factors. Manipulation of instruments should be careful and slow, and the cervical preparation described above may also reduce the risk. A clear vision is mandatory especially when dissection or energy is being considered.

It is important to recognize a uterine perforation—there is loss of resistance in the manipulation of the instruments, loss of distension of the endometrial cavity, rapid increase in fluid deficit, and possible visualization of the pelvic organs as intestine or adipose tissue. Other suggestive signs may include excessive bleeding, hypotension, and acute hematuria. The approach to uterine perforation depends on the instrument used, the size, and location of the perforation. General measures include removal of all instruments and assessment of the patient's hemodynamic status, as well as abdominal and pelvic examination.[4]

Fundal and axial perforations, without the use of an energy source, can usually be approached conservatively. The patient should be monitored and kept under surveillance. If stable, patient may be discharged and should be aware about warning signs (pain, fever, bloating, and bleeding). In other locations, additional measures may be required:
- In low anterior perforations, if there is concern regarding possible bladder injury, the integrity of the structures can be tested through the administration of contrast or cystoscopy can be performed.
- Lateral perforations may involve the broad ligament, ureters, and large pelvic vessels; posterior perforations may involve the rectum; perforations with sharp curettes or electrosurgical instruments may originate lacerations or burns. In these cases, laparoscopy (preferred) or laparotomy (usually reserved for hemodynamically unstable patients) is warranted. If bowel injury is suspected, the support of General Surgery should be requested, since it is difficult to assess the integrity of the entire bowel by laparoscopy. Depending on the site of the injury, support from urology or vascular surgery may also be requested.[5]
- If occult hemorrhage is suspected, analyses (blood count and coagulation) and pelvic ultrasound should be performed to look for hematoma. If there are complaints of abdominal or shoulder pain, diagnostic laparoscopy is indicated.[1]

Prophylactic antibiotic therapy is not mandatory in uncomplicated uterine perforations. The use of antibiotics is only indicated in complicated perforations or with signs of infection.

False Route

It occurs when the hysteroscope enters the muscle fibers, rather than progressing into the intrauterine cavity through the internal cervical orifice. In this situation, the cervical muscle fibers are visualized, instead of the triangular cavity and bilateral ostia. To prevent this complication, cervical dilation should be careful; ideally, the entrance should be done with vaginoscopy, with direct visualization and slow entry into the cervical canal. Previously described cervical ripening methods may also help.

Faced with the creation of a false path, the instrument must be carefully removed. If the diagnosis of false path is confirmed, in most cases the procedure should be discontinued, as this complication carries a higher risk of volume overload due to excessive fluid absorption. Some authors advocate that the procedure can be continued, but the data are insufficient to demonstrate its safety.[5]

Cervical Laceration

It can occur particularly in cases of cervical stenosis. Cervical lacerations can be associated with significant bleeding (point out that lateral lacerations can reach the uterine arteries!). The approach to lacerations includes compression of the affected area; in case of persistence of bleeding, hemostatic agents (Monsel's solution) or diathermy may be used. If large or very bleeding, they should be sutured.[3,5]

Vasovagal Reaction

Most often it is related to acute severe pain, usually during dilation and/or entry into the cervical canal or during uterine distension. Signs and symptoms include a prodrome with pallor, diaphoresis, nausea/vomiting followed by hypotension and bradycardia. The procedure should be suspended, put the patient in supine position with elevated legs or in Trendelenburg position and evaluate vital signs. Most vasovagal reactions resolve with these measures. Otherwise, support from the resuscitation team should be sought, as there may be a need for administration of intravenous fluids or even atropine.[1,5]

Hemorrhage

When resection procedures are performed or when complications such as cervical laceration/uterine perforation occur, there may be considerable bleeding. The intracavitary fluid pressure itself leads to the collapse of the vessels and helps control bleeding. In most cases, intrauterine hemorrhage is controllable by electrocoagulation, but this does not always happen when it comes to larger vessels. If there is refractory or diffuse bleeding, the procedure should be stopped; the hypothesis of coagulopathy should be evaluated and coagulation tests ordered; therapeutic alternatives in these cases include bimanual compression, use of intravenous tranexamic acid, intracervical injection of vasopressin, placement of an inflated Foley catheter balloon (20–30 cc saline) into the endometrial cavity. In cases refractory to these measures, consider uterine embolization or even emergent hysterectomy.[1]

LATE UTERINE COMPLICATIONS

Among the late complications, intrauterine adhesions and infection stand out.[3]

Intrauterine Adhesions

The appearance of intrauterine adhesions depends on the procedure performed. They are more common after myomectomies, endometrial ablation, and metroplasty. They may manifest as hematometra, amenorrhea, pelvic pain, or dysmenorrhea due to retrograde menstruation. Prevention is important, especially in women of childbearing age. If there is indication for myomectomies in opposite uterine walls, this can be performed in two times, to prevent the formation of adhesions. Other preventive measures are the use of mechanical barriers, such as an intrauterine balloon (e.g., Foley catheter), intrauterine device, or hormonal therapy (estrogens and progestogen).[3]

Infection

Postoperative infections are rare; they include cystitis, endometritis, pyometra, and pelvic inflammatory disease (PID).[3] If pelvic infection is suspected or in patients with risk factors, treatment should be undertaken prior to hysteroscopy. In the absence of suspicion of pelvic infectious pathology, as post-hysteroscopy infection is rare, prophylactic antibiotic therapy is not generally indicated.[1] An exception to this might be the coexistence of tubal disease or endometriosis.

COMPLICATION RELATED TO ANESTHESIA

Most patients who undergo diagnostic or surgical hysteroscopy with a simple procedure (such as

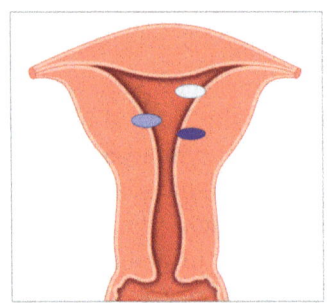
Degree of penetration of the myoma into myometrium

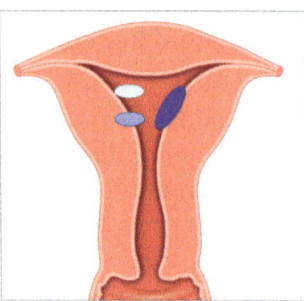
The extension of the base of the nodule with respect to the wall of the uterus

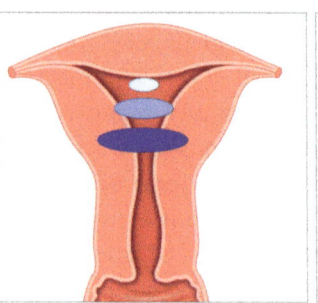
Size of the nodule: Up to 2 cm, between 2 and 5 cm and more than 5 cm

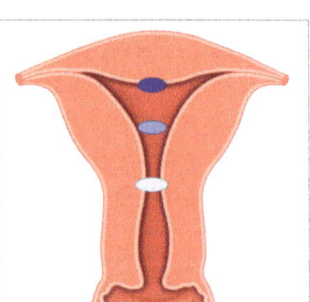
Topography: In the lateral wall an extra point is added

		Size (cm)	Topography	Extension of the base	Penetration	Lateral wall	Total
STEPW classification	0	<2	Low	<1/3	0	+1	
	1	2 to 5	Middle	1/3 to 2/3	<50%		
	2	>5	Upper	>2/3	>50%		

	Score	Group	Complexity and therapeutic options
○ = Score 0	0 to 4	I	Low complexity hysteroscopic myomectomy
◐ = Score 1	5 to 6	II	High complexity hysteroscopic myomectomy. Consider GnRH use. Consider two-step hysteroscopic myomectomy
● = Score 2	7 to 9	III	Consider alternatives to the hysteroscopic technique

Fig. 1: STEPW classification. (GnRH: gonadotropin hormone-releasing hormone)
Courtesy: Hysteroscopy Newsletter

polypectomies or myomectomy) do not require anesthesia. If the pain associated with the examination is not tolerated, paracervical/intracervical block may be considered.

As office hysteroscopy is quite common, the gynecologist should be aware of the complications related to the use of local anesthetics. Toxicity occurs when there is unintentional intravascular administration or administration of toxic doses. To prevent this complication, aspiration should be done before injecting to ensure that the topical anesthetic is not injected directly into a vessel.

Clinical manifestations of toxicity usually include cardiac and neurological symptoms. Initial symptoms include metallic taste, perioral paresthesia, agitation, dysarthria, hypertension, tachycardia, and arrhythmias, progressing to seizures, bradycardia, and asystole. If toxicity is suspected, the procedure should be suspended, the resuscitation team should be called, the patient should be monitored (including cardiac monitoring) and intravenous accesses should be placed.[5]

COMPLICATION RELATED TO SURGEON

Of course, operator experience is essential when it comes to complications. On the one hand, dexterity, and on the other hand, the experience that allows to evaluate when to continue or stop a procedure are essential especially in the most difficult cases.

Regarding myomectomy, in 2005, the STEPW classification was developed to evaluate the feasibility and difficulty of hysteroscopic myomectomy. This classification considers the degree of penetration of the myoma into the myometrium, the distance of the base of the myoma from the uterine wall, the size of the nodule, and the topography of the uterine cavity. The total score allows for a better planning of the surgery **(Fig. 1)**.[6]

CONCLUSION

To conclude, a safe procedure is dependent on preoperative assessment of the patient, the choice of the right instruments, and sometimes previous cervical preparation and of course the expertise of the surgeon and his awareness to identify complications, manage them, and, when necessary, stop the procedure.

REFERENCES

1. Hoffman BL, Schorge JO, Halvorson LM, Hamid CA, Corton MM, Schaffer JI. Williams Gynecology, 4th edition. New York: McGraw Hill; 2020.
2. ACOG Committee. The Use of Hysteroscopy for the Diagnosis and Treatment of Intrauterine Pathology: ACOG Committee Opinion, Number 800. Obstet Gynecol. 2020;135(3):e138-e148.
3. Nabi S. Hysteroscopic Complications. Eur J Med Health Sci. 2022;4(3):13-6.
4. Elahmedawy H, Snook NJ. Complications of operative hysteroscopy: an anaesthetist's perspective. BJA Edu. 2021;21(7):240-2.
5. Serranito A. (2023). Operative Hysteroscopy Complications. [online] Available from: https://www.intechopen.com/chapters/85288. [Last accessed November, 2023].
6. Lasmar RB, Barrozo PR, Dias R, Oliveira MA. Submucous myomas: a new presurgical classification to evaluate the viability of hysteroscopic surgical treatment—preliminary report. J Minim Invasive Gynecol. 2005;12(4):308-11.

Chapter 19: Practical Tips in Operative Hysteroscopy

Osama Shawki

INTRODUCTION

Hysteroscopy is an amazing technology. Though it looks simple, this surgery is difficult. We need proper visualization and follow time limit means intrauterine surgery to be completed in time limit. The common pathologies we come across in day-to-day practice are polyp, submucous myoma, intrauterine adhesions, and uterine septum. The success of surgery depends upon many factors such as good visualization with proper distension and adequate light source. With perfect instruments, we require diamond tips always. Let us learn few important facts.

How to maintain good view at hysteroscopy uterine distension?

- The greatest challenge in hysteroscopy is to keep good view and maintain good distension throughout the procedure. Without good distension, you can never put correct diagnosis neither perform operative procedure. There are many recommendations and advices from experts and textbooks. You can never standardize fixed pressure that suits every uterus.
- The postmenopausal small uterus may be well distended by lower pressure, whereas a multiparous large size uterus will demand higher pressure to keep uterine cavity distended. Thus, it is quite variable.
- You should step up pressure till you get enough to keep uterine walls apart and cavity distended allowing proper panoramic view. Pressure should not be higher than mean arterial pressure for long time, as this will push much fluid into circulation and put the patient at risk of fluid overload.
- For office and simple diagnostic procedures, you may use gravity pressure or cuff-driven pressure. However, for longer operative procedure, a fluid pump is essential, preferably to measure the inflow outflow volume. If the deficit is approaching 1 L, then you must stop and abandon the procedure.
- In cases with wide patulous cervix and lot of fluid escape, you may apply a tenaculum at angle of external os to squeeze the hysteroscopy sheath and avoid leakage of fluid.
- For good vaginoscopy, your assistance should be trained to close the vaginal outlet so that vagina gets properly distended to perform vaginal surgeries.

KNOW YOUR INSTRUMENTS

- Proper alignments and careful handling is very important. Everyone should have at least 2.9-mm hysteroscope with inner and outer sheath. With 2.9-mm hysteroscope and 5-French scissors, forceps, and bipolar electrode, we can deal with many problems such as polyp and septum intrauterine adhesions.
- We can negotiate the small pinhole ostium with water pressure, forceps, and scissors. When we open the blades of scissors, the distance is 6 mm and when we open the jaws of forceps, the distance is 8 mm. So while negotiating the narrow cavity, one should open the forceps or scissors to move forward. The movements should be gentle and precise.
- While using electrosurgical unit, never push with current on. Have a practice of moving loop, all directions.
- Use pressure pump systems and do proper settings. Learn your instrument and set it properly with pressure and inflow per minute with bar.

TIPS AND TRICKS FOR POLYPS

- *Tip 1*: There are two methods—with forceps and with scissors. For small polyps, one can use forceps. Grasp the polyp at the base and remove it by push technique.

Try to measure the polyp by simple opening the jaws of forceps. When we use scissor, always make sure that you cut the polyp at exact base and avoid getting superficial part leaving base of polyp. Not to go deep into myometrium as it will cause pain at office procedure.
- *Tip 2*: For anterior wall polyp, always lower your hands down to direct the scissors into upward and forward direction and target base of polyp. For posterior wall polyp, you do vice versa.
- *Tip 3*: The challenge and difficulty is in the lateral wall and cornual polyps, where the direction of telescope is not toward that angle. It is impossible to move the hysteroscope at right angle to reach that angular polyp on side walls. In that case, you should rotate the telescope so as the scissors blade will point toward lateral wall and can easily access polyp.
- *Tip 4*: Scissors are preferred for small polyps, but resectoscope will be better for larger polyps to cut into pieces and allow easy extraction.
- *Tip 5*: If polyp is cut and cannot be extracted, you may leave it but take the biopsy. You may give patient misoprostol to stimulate uterine contractions. The polyp will be spontaneously extruded shortly.

UTERINE SEPTUM: DIAMOND TIPS

- *Tip 1*: There was controversy among many people that septum is an additional tissue, which should be excised, resected, and removed to restore normal shape of uterus. From observation of hysteroscopic septum division, we notice that once you cut into central part of septum, the tissues retract and fly back to anterior and posterior wall of uterus. There are no residual tissues of septum after cutting it. This brings the fact that septum tissues are part of anterior and posterior wall of uterine muscles, which became fused in central part of cavity. Once you incise and divide it, it retracts and is released back to be incorporated in the uterine walls. So, the key message is that septum is never resected neither removed. Simply, hysteroscopic division results in the release of septal fibers and allows its retraction to fill and strengthen uterine walls. The view of uterine cavity after completion of septum surgery is very typical. It clearly shows pinkish colored area towards cornu and at the center white triangle that is the septum bed. Shortly the endometrium creeps and heals this white surface resulting complete unification two cavities covering the new added triangular space of the septum scar. In that sense, it is augmentation hysteroplasty.
- *Tip 2:* For a long time, people used to think of septum as mostly fibrous element and scarce in vascularity. Recent research proved beyond doubt that septum is combined muscular and fibrous tissue with predominance of muscular element. Moreover, it is very rich in vascular channels. If you observe the video of septum division, you will realize obviously that the lower most part starting at cervix is more fibrous, but the more we climb up toward the fundus, the muscular component become more predominant. Also, it is obvious that the central part of septum is richly vascular, while the lateral edges harbor more fibrous components.
- *Tip 3:* Choice between scissors or electrosurgery for septum division is a very frequent enquiry from colleagues. My recommendation is to use the scissors for the thinner septum however long it is. But for the wide base broad septum, you will need electrosurgery. Bipolar is much safer to avoid the possible threat of fluid overload and electrolyte imbalance. You can start with 2.9-mm office hysteroscope then open the blades of scissors and judge the septum and then plan cautery if septum is thick.
- *Tip 4:* Timing for procedure: According to the general rule, all hysteroscopic procedures are preferably performed in early proliferative phase where endometrium is thin and not obstructing vision. But if we are suspecting tuberculosis then the best time for conducting hysteroscopic examination is premenstrual phase so that any overlying deposits are not missed out.

  However, preoperative combined OCP for two cycles may be enough to induce thin endometrium and improve the field of vision during surgery.
- Do we need a concomitant laparoscopy control during hysteroscopic septum division? The answer is definitely No. Laparoscopic control will tell you once transillumination of hysteroscopy light starts to appear. Then, this means you already cut too far into fundus myometrium. The best control in case you need it is concomitant abdominal ultrasound to measure thickness of fundus and judge limit to stop.
- *Tip 5:* Do we need postoperative barrier method like intrauterine contraceptive device (IUCD) or balloon after septum surgery? The answer is No. Insertion of foreign material may add risk of infection and adhesion

formation. In fact, the healthy endometrium in each cornu will grow and creep easily to cover the surface of septum bed. Addition of estrogen replacement might help despite not needed in most instances.
- *Tip 6*: When to allow pregnancy and mode of delivery? Hysteroscopic division leaves no myometrial scar. Pregnancy can be allowed after three cycles and mode of delivery can be normal unless other indication for C-section.
- *Tip 7*: A frequently asked question; How may I develop my skills in septum surgery? My advice is that you should start by picking cases of short and thin septum to practice for scissors maneuvering and orientation of cavity properly. Once you master the scissors job, then you can start the electrosurgery technique.

MYOMA RESECTION: DIAMOND TIPS

- *Tip 1:* Always do good ultrasound and preferably 3D, i.e., mapping to assess the degree of myoma bulge into cavity. Proper myoma mapping is very important to plan the surgery.
- *Tip 2:* Bigger myoma should be avoided or planned on two sessions. Patient's counseling should be done.
- *Tip 3:* Bipolar resection under saline distention fluid is much safer to avoid fluid overload and hyponatremia complications.
- *Tip 4:* The golden rule in myoma resection is to maintain good distention, panoramic clear view, and enough space between myoma and uterine wall. This will allow safe and controlled resection without injury to adjacent endometrium.
- *Tip 5:* For larger myoma, you may start resection from both sides. It should be like eating apple taking bite from each side and convert the ball shape myoma into small banana shape. Afterwards, the residual central banana shape piece is grasped and twisted out of uterus.
- *Tip 6:* If myoma has considerable intramural part, try to find the plane between myoma and myometrium by cutting circumferentially. Then dissect the fibers and try to enucleate from its base gently as we do laparoscopically. Or you can remove it in next setting. Sometimes once you reached this level, the fluid pressure will help to deliver and push the myoma from its deep bed and make it bulge further into cavity. The more experience you develop, the more possibility you can deal with deeper myomas.

- *Tip 7:* For smaller myoma, scissors release form base and enucleation is feasible as office procedure. Careful dissection should reach the layer between myoma and myometrium, then procedure will run easy and smooth afterward.
- *Tip 8:* Extraction of resected pieces can be done under vision using the electrode to catch and extract pieces. A tissue forceps can also help but will not be able to catch all pieces. An alternative easy technique is to use a large caliber suction cannula for evacuation of uterus. Adding misoprostol for 5 days postoperative will help to complete expulsion for residual pieces.

INTRAUTERINE ADHESIONS (ASHERMAN SYNDROME): DIAMOND TIPS

- *Tip 1:* If possible plan good hysterosalpingography (HSG). HSG is your map and GPS to give directions and exact plan for hysteroscopic release of adhesions.
- *Tip 2:* Use the smallest diameter hysteroscope and preferably the office set. The Asherman cavity is already restricted in size and dimensions. It will be difficult if you attempt using larger sheath.
- *Tip 3:* Avoid using electrosurgery in Asherman reconstruction. The uterus has already very scanty endometrium. The use of electrosurgery to release adhesions will eventually destroy whatever residual endometrium she has. Also, the regeneration power of cauterized tissues will be very weak and limited.
- *Tip 4:* Scissors is more preferred than anything else.
- *Tip 5:* In cases when adhesions at lower segment and obstructing access to cavity, the sheath will not be able to go deep enough the cavity. Consequently, there will be lot of leakage of distension fluid and inability to maintain good distension of cervical canal. In that case, follow the golden tip by applying a single tooth tenaculum on the angle of cervix at 3 or 9 o'clock to squeeze tightly the hysteroscopy sheath and avoid leakage of fluid. Additional advantage to that tip is that the high distension pressure will exert push on the isthmic adhesions and put it under tension and tenting. That will facilitate identification for the weakest point and start release of adhesions. Something like imperforate Hymen bulging by pressure of hematocolpos.
- *Tip 6:* Hysterography under fluoroscopy during reconstruction might help in identification of limit and degree of expansion of uterus. Also, concomitant

ultrasound is helpful. Laparoscopy will not add much information.
- *Tip 7:* Always counsel the patient that the procedure might need to be redone several times till it achieves good size cavity.
- *Tip 8:* Always search for a landmark like tubal ostium to start release of adhesions in directions based on proper anatomical identification.
- *Tip 9:* Insertion of physical barrier like Folly's balloon catheter is a must. It should be left for at least 7–9 days with sequential estrogen therapy for at least three cycles then second look for evaluation.
- One can use hyaluronic acid gel after surgery which is very important part of connective tissue. It will help in healing.
- *Tip 10:* If patient get pregnant, be prepared for possibility of placenta accrete.

CONCLUSION

Hysteroscopy is amazing intrauterine technology. Though it looks simple, there are many troubleshootings. Adequate and appropriate instrumentations, proper knowledge of the pathology, patient and preparation, expertise, understanding all the tips and tricks will give you wonderful results.

INDEX

Page numbers followed by *f* refer to figure and *t* refer to table.

A

Abdomen 78
Abnormal uterine bleeding 19, 55, 80
  evaluation of 2
Abortion, surgical 76
Acetic acid 84
Acidic vaginal environment 85
Acute respiratory distress syndrome 14
Adenocarcinoma, endometrial 92
Adenoma, juvenile cystic 41
Adiana matrix 98*f*
Admirable rewarding technology 1
American Fertility Society 29, 45
American Society for Reproductive
    Medicine 29, 30, 35, 37*f*, 45, 45*t*
  features of 30*t*
Analgesia 19
Ancillary instruments 38*f*
Anesthesia 104
Antibiotic prophylaxis 73
Anxiety 19
Asherman's cavity 108
Asherman's syndrome 21*f*, 45, 64, 108
Assisted reproductive technique 59
Atrophic endometrium 92*f*, 93
Atropine 19
Autoclave sterilization 12
Auto-cross-linked hyaluronic acid gel 50
Automated fluid pump 15, 16*f*

B

Basal cells 85
Bettocchi integrated office hysteroscope
    telescope 20*f*
Bipolar electrode 10, 17, 106
  needle 34*f*, 47, 48*f*
Bipolar energy 17
Bipolar hook electrode 18*f*
Bipolar resectoscope 17, 17*f*, 18*f*
  use of 100*f*
Bipolar system 17
Bipolar versapoint electrodes 10
Bizarre dirty endometrium 62*f*
Bleeding, postmenopausal 92, 93
Blunt cervical canal 61*f*
Bone fragments 80*f*
Bowel lesion 101
Broken Karman cannula tip 80*f*

C

Camera
  connecting unit 20
  system 2

Cancer, endometrial 2, 93
Carbon dioxide 13
Carcinoma 93
  endometrial 94, 94*f*
Cervical
  agenesis 35
  canal 61, 66*f*, 68*f*, 79*f*, 81
  dilatation 21
  ectopic pregnancy 100
    diagnosis of 100
    management of 100
  fibroids 56
  laceration 101, 103
  orifice
    external 61
    internal 61
  pathology, evaluation of 97
  uterine junction 66*f*
Cervix 40, 60, 66*f*, 95, 97
  double 33*f*, 95
  evaluation of 96
Cesarean scar 66*f*, 95
  defect 66, 70*f*
Chlamydia 59
  trachomatis 59
Chromopertubation 42*f*, 64
CO_2 tubal insufflator 16, 16*f*
Collin's knife 11*f*, 33*f*, 48
Collin's loop 57*f*
Conception
  early 77
  retained products of 19, 76, 77, 77*f*
Contiguous cells 84
Cord, clear stricture of 99*f*
Cyst, inclusion 67*f*
Cystic lesion 42*f*

D

Diabetes mellitus 24
Diode laser 26*f*
Distension media 2, 9, 13, 102
  characteristics of 14*t*
  types of 9, 13

E

Eastman theory 76
Ectopic gestational sac 99*f*
Ectopic pregnancy 72, 95, 99
  extraction of 100*f*
  hysteroscopic removal of 99
Edema, pulmonary 14
Electrodes 3, 10
  loop of 77
  needle 25

Electronic suction and irrigation pump 9
Electrosurgical injury 101
Electrosurgical unit 3, 13, 16
Embryofetoscopy 98, 99
Embryoscopy 95
Endocervical scarring 63
Endochondral ossification 80
Endometrial cavity 42*f*, 43*f*
Endometrial mucosa, inflammation of 59
Endometrial thickness 93
Endometriosis 72
  development of 42
Endometritis 59, 104
Endometrium 50, 60, 63*f*, 79, 94
  guide pockets of 49
  hyperemic 63*f*
Endoscopes 5
  types of 5
Energy
  types of 13
  use of 48
Epithelial progenitor cells 51
Essure device, coil of 98*f*
Estrogen 24
  exogenous 93
European Society for Gynaecological
    Endoscopy 29, 30, 31*f*, 54
  classification 54*f*, 54*t*
  features of 30
European Society of Human Reproduction
    and Embryology 29, 30, 31*f*
  features of 30*t*

F

Fallopian tube 60, 75*f*
  diseases 72
Female genital tuberculosis, hormone
    dependent nature of 60
Female reproductive system, developmental
    malformations of 35
Fertility evaluation 39
Fiber optic cable 88
Fibroids 53
  lateral wall 54
Fibrosis 62*f*
Fibrotic tissue 61*f*, 68*f*
  resection of 70*f*
  thickened 62*f*
Fluid 102
  absorption 14
  distension media 13
  high-viscosity 14
  intravasation 101
  overload 14, 15, 102

Fluoroscopic guidance 49
Fluoroscopy 108
    unit 73
Foley's catheter 33*f*
    pediatric 49

G

Gas 102
    embolism 101, 102
    sterilization 12
Genital organs 60
Genital tuberculosis 60, 64
Gestational sac, opening of 98*f*
Glycine 9
    toxicity 15
Gonadotropin releasing hormone 15, 54, 104*f*
Gonorrhea 59
Granulomas 63
Grasper 25
Gravitation system 15*f*
Gutenberg classification 76

H

Halogen 8
Hamou's microcolpoisteroscope, types of 86*f*
Hamou's microhysteroscope 5
Hegar's dilator 82
Hellman theory 76
Hematometra 43*f*, 46
Hemorrhage 101, 103
Hemostatic resection, twizzle tip for 18
High-frequency angled ball electrode 69
Hopkins hysteroscope 5
Hormone therapy 50
Hyaluronic acid 49
Hyperemia 60, 63*f*
Hyperplasia 92
    complex 94
    endometrial 55, 92*f*, 93
    simple 94
Hypertension 24
Hyponatremia, dilution 15
Hypotheses, several 66
Hysterography 108
Hysteromat 10*f*, 20*f*
Hysterosalpingogram 73, 75*f*
Hysterosalpingography 24, 35, 46
Hysteroscope 1*f*, 5*f*, 38*f*, 39*f*, 68, 73
    flexible 6
    philosophy of 1
Hysteroscopic
    adhesiolysis 48*f*, 49
    cannulation 42*f*
    grasper 11*f*, 82, 82*f*
        forceps 82
    isthmocele appearance 70*f*
    isthmoplasty 68*f*
    metroplasty 29, 69
    morcellator 10, 11*f*
    myomectomy 53, 54*f*
        complexity of 56
    scissors 11*f*, 47, 98*f*
    surgery, majority of 38
    tissue removal system 22*f*, 24, 25, 27*f*
    treatment, flattening effect of 68*f*
Hysteroscopy 1, 2, 13, 14*t*, 15, 24, 25*f*, 35, 38*f*, 43*f*, 55, 55*f*, 59-61, 64, 76, 76*t*, 92, 95, 101, 106
    advantage of 64, 77
    diagnosis 93
    expanded scope of 95-99
    indications for 2
    instruments for 5
    irrigation fluid 7*f*
    modern development of 95
    office 105
    operative 16, 106
    role of 35
    smart use of 66
    unit, set up of 2
    use of 96*f*
    uterine distension 106
    virtual 46
Hysterosonography 55
Hysterotomy closure, nonabsorbable suture for 80

I

In situ intrauterine contraceptive device 81*f*
Infection 101, 104
Infertility 72, 73, 80
    evaluation of 2
Inflammation, intrauterine 80
Instruments
    maintenance of 12
    sterilization of 12
Intermittent balloon dilatation, use of 51*f*
International Federation of Gynecology and Obstetrics myoma classification 54*f*
Intracervical vasopressin 15
Intramural fibroids 55
Intrauterine adhesions 45, 46*f*, 48*f*, 101, 104, 108
    American Fertility Society classification of 45
    American Society for Reproductive Medicine classification of 45*t*
Intrauterine
    balloon stent 49, 49*f*
    contraceptive device 22*f*, 49, 78, 79, 79*f*, 81*f*
        in situ 79*f*
    pressure, low 15
    sutures, retained 80
Irregular pale endometrium 63*f*
Irrigation bag 10*f*
Isotonic electrolyte-containing solutions 14
Isotonic fluid media 15
Isthmocele 66-68, 68*f*
    basic measurements of 67*f*
    hysteroscopic appearance 67*f*
    site 66*f*
Isthmoplasty, hysteroscopic 68*f*

J

Jacques Hamou's microcolpohysteroscope 84

K

Karman's cannula, retrieved broken tip of 82*f*
Koilocyte 85*f*
Koilocytosis 85, 90*f*

L

Laminaria tent 79
Laser 25
Lasmar classification 54, 54*f*, 54*t*
Leiomyoma 18*f*
Lippes loop, misplaced 78*f*
Liquid
    crystal display monitors 9
    distension medium 38
Loop electrode 11*f*
Lugol's solution 84, 88*f*
    application of 97*f*

M

Manual pressure system 15, 16*f*
Mature superficial squamous epithelium 97*f*
Mechanical tissue retrieval system 77, 77*f*
Menopause 93*t*
Menorrhagia 79
Menstrual drainage 68*f*
Mesenchymal cells 51
Metal cannula, broken tip of 83*f*
Methylene blue test 32*f*
Metroplasty, hysteroscopic 29, 69
Microcatheter 73
Microcolpohysteroscopy 86*f*-90*f*, 97*f*
Microhysteroscope 7
Micropolyps 60
    hysteroscopic picture of 60*f*
Mini Gubbini resectoscope 22*f*
Miniature hysteroscopes, application of 47
Mini-hysteroresectoscope 68*f*
Mini-resectoscope 25, 48*f*, 69*f*
Misoprostol 19
Monopolar electrodes 10
Monopolar resectoscope 17*f*
Müllerian agenesis 35

Index

Müllerian anomalies 35, 46, 95
   American Society for Reproductive Medicine classification of 37*f*
   diagnosis of 35
   nonseptate 35
Müllerian malformations 38
Multiload CuT, misplaced broken arm of 82*f*
Mycobacterium tuberculosis 60
Mycoplasma hominis 59
Myoma 18*f*
   enucleation 57*f*
   intramural penetration of 54
   resection 108
Myomectomy 5, 19, 57
   ambulatory 56
   hysteroscopic 53, 54*f*
   low complexity hysteroscopic 54
   office 56
Myometrial closure technique 66
Myometrial thickness, adjacent 67
Myometrium 54
   residual 68*f*

N

Neisseria gonorrhoeae 59
Neodymium-doped yttrium aluminum garnet 25
Niche, proximal rim of 68*f*
Nodule's diameter 57
Nonseptate Müllerian duct anomalies, management of 35
No-touch hysteroscopy 95
Novy catheter 74*f*

O

Obesity 24
Office hysteroscopy 4, 19, 105
   indications for 19
   smart tips for 22
Office myomectomy 56
Oliguria 14
Osseous metaplasia 22*f*, 79, 80*f*
Osseous tissue, removal of 82
Ostia polyp 26*f*
Ovabloc intra tubal device 97
Ovaries 60

P

Pain 78
Parabasal cells 85
Partial septum 32*f*
   hysteroscopic view of 32*f*, 34*f*
Pediatric Foleys bulb in situ 50*f*
Pelvic
   examination 80
   infectious pathology 104
   inflammatory disease 72, 78, 104
   magnetic resonance imaging of 42*f*
   pain, chronic 73, 78
   ultrasonography 24
Periodic acid-Schiff reagent 85
Plasma volume 14
Polypectomy, hysteroscopic 24, 27*f*
Polyps 55, 92-94, 106, 107
   anterior wall 107
   asymptomatic 24
   base of 26*f*
   cornual 107
   diagnosis of 24
   endometrial 24, 93
   single sessile 25*f*
   small 19
   symptomatic 24
   treatment of 24
Postintervention fertility evaluation 74
Power Doppler 24
Pregnancy, medical termination of 80
Pressure
   cuff 9
   system 13, 106
Proximal tubal
   cannulation 72, 74
   occlusion 72
      assessment 73
      etiology of 72
Pseudopolypoid endometrium 60
Pyometra 104

R

Ranney theory 76
Rectovaginal septum, endometriosis of 96*f*
Renal failure, acute 14
Reproductive system 35
Resectoscope 3, 8, 25
   parts of 8*f*
Rigid hysteroscope 5, 20*f*, 38
Robert's uterus 41
Rollerball electrode 11*f*
Royal College of Obstetricians and Gynaecologists 29

S

Saline
   infusion sonogram 46
   sonohysterography 73
Salpingitis isthmica nodosa 72
Second look hysteroscopy 19
Semi-rigid versascope system 6
Septal resection 21*f*, 43*f*
Septate uterus, complete 32*f*
Septum 32*f*
   complete 32*f*, 33*f*, 39
   partial 32*f*
Small diameter resectoscope 68
Sonohysterography 24
Sorbitol toxicity 15
Squamocolumnar junction 84, 85*f*, 89*f*, 97*f*
Squamocylindrical junction 84
Squamous intraepithelial lesion, high-grade 90*f*
Standard Bettocchi hysteroscope 5
Starry sky appearance 64
Stem cell 51, 85
Stenotic cervix 19
STEPW classification 104*f*
Sterilization, intrauterine 97
Strawberry appearance 60
Stromal cells 51
Subcylindrical reserve cells 85
Submucosal fibroids 54
   classification of 54
   diagnosis of 55
Submucous myoma 53, 56*f*
   classification 53
   types 53
   vision of 55*f*
Subserosal myoma 55*f*
Suction cannula, broken tip of 82
Surgery, intrauterine 13
Surgical hysteroscopy
   complications of 38
   instrumentation of 38
Synechiae 63

T

Tamoxifen 24
Tissue, endometrial 51
Toxicity, clinical manifestations of 105
Transvaginal sonography 2
Transvaginal ultrasound 32*f*, 67*f*, 93
Transverse vaginal septum 35, 40
T-shaped uterus 40
   narrow cavity of 40*f*
Tubal blockages 72
Tubal cannulation
   instruments, complete set of 74*f*
   hysteroscopic visualization of 74*f*
Tubal occlusion, bilateral 75*f*
Tubal ostia 73
Tubal ostial fibrosis 63
Tubal ostium 42*f*, 98
Tubal sterilization 95
Tubal surgery, previous 72
Tubercle 61*f*, 63*f*
Tuberculosis 59, 60
   endometrial 60
   endometritis 21*f*
   genital 60, 64
Twizzle electrode 10*f*

U

Ulceration 64
Ultrasonography 60, 76, 76*t*
   transrectal 42*f*

Ultrasound
    forceps extraction 79
    guided radiofrequency ablation 57
Umbilical cord
    stricture 98f
    visualization of 99f
Urology stone grasper 82f
Uterine
    adnexa, investigation of 55
    anomalies
        European Society for Gynaecological Endoscopy classification of 31f
        European Society of Human Reproduction and Embryology classification of 31f
    bleeding, postmenopausal 92, 93t
    cavity 35, 42f, 43, 43f, 55, 68f, 73, 78, 78f, 79f, 81, 87f, 88f, 92
        evaluation of 39
        hysteroscopic illumination of 43f
        multilayered squamous epithelium of 84f
        normal 40f, 97f
        pathological microscopic aspects of 84
        view of 64f
    complications, late 104
    fundus 32f
    lateral wall 81f
    leiomyomas 53
    malformations
        congenital 29
        hysteroscopic surgery of 38
    mass, accessory cavitated 41
    perforation 30, 101, 102
    polyp 21f
    septum 29, 42f, 43f, 107
        asymmetric 43f
        normal fundus after excision of 43f
        postexcision of 43f
        pre-excision of 43
    structure, external 35
    wall 54
        thickness 31f, 32f
Uterotubal ostium 72
Uterus 1f
    bicornuate 35, 41, 41f
    didelphys 35
    magnetic resonance imaging of 55f
    philosophy of 1
    postmenopausal small 106
    right cornual part of 42f
    septate 35
    T-shaped 40
    unicornuate 35, 41, 41f

V

Vacuum aspiration 79
Vagina 60, 95f
Vaginal canal, distension of 95
Vaginal discharge, offensive 78
Vaginal pathology 95
Vaginal polyp 26f
Vaginal repair 69
Vaginal septum 33f, 95
    longitudinal 35
Vaginal speculum 85
Vaginitis 96f
Vaginoscopy 95, 95f, 96, 96f
Vascular flow 50
Vasovagal reaction 101, 103
Versascope 6f
Vessels, coagulation of 100f
Visceral bladder 101
Vulva 60

W

Waterman's blue ink 84
Womb 1

X

Xenon 8

www.ingramcontent.com/pod-product-compliance
Ingram Content Group UK Ltd.
Pitfield, Milton Keynes, MK11 3LW, UK
UKHW052230140425
457402UK00006B/35